BEYOND KISSINGER:
WAYS OF CONSERVATIVE STATECRAFT

Studies in International Affairs Number 26

Also by George Liska

International Equilibrium

Nations in Alliance: The Limits of Interdependence

Imperial America: The International Politics of Primacy

States in Evolution: Changing Societies and Traditional Systems in World Politics

Studies in International Affairs Number 26

BEYOND KISSINGER: WAYS
OF CONSERVATIVE STATECRAFT

George Liska

*The Washington Center of
Foreign Policy Research
School of Advanced International Studies
The Johns Hopkins University*

*The Johns Hopkins University Press
Baltimore and London*

Manufactured in the United States of America.

The Johns Hopkins University Press, Baltimore, Maryland 21218
The Johns Hopkins University Press Ltd., London

Library of Congress Catalog Card Number 75–10838
ISBN 0–8018–1763–3 (clothbound edition)
ISBN 0–8018–1764–1 (paperbound edition)

Library of Congress Cataloging in Publication data will be found on the last printed page of this book.

For Suzy

CONTENTS

PREFACE

As this manuscript is being surrendered to the publisher, the international situation is once again highly fluid and replete with crosscurrents. The most perverse consequences of actions and developments are the most probable ones. Thus, the catastrophe in Indochina affected American diplomacy in the Middle East in one way when doubts about U.S. commitments stiffened Israel's reluctance to give up territorial security assets in exchange for pledges underwritten by the United States. It may affect the situation in the Middle East in another way, reinforcing Israel's resolve and nullifying the administration's instinct for reprisal, if determination to verify America's reliability as an ally and offset Soviet gains in Southeast Asia converts retaliation against Israeli "intransigence" into stronger-than-ever support for Israeli "firmness." As a result, world-wide détente with the Soviet Union would be transformed into confrontation in the Middle East by way of the collapse in Indochina, just as transient conciliation in Southeast Asia (in 1972–73) had previously instigated the most recent and far-reaching spell of détente. An American-Soviet confrontation in a theater still relatively favorable to the United States—if more in domestic than in military-strategic terms—might undo some, at least, of the Soviets' discreetly appreciated successes in Vietnam as well as in Western Europe (Portugal) and the Middle East (the "movement" toward Geneva and, possibly, toward matching and even reversing the solely American prior access to both local sides). The cause-effect chain would then be nearly as involved as was that between Soviet support for the OPEC policy of oil embargo and price-rise and the late drift of a previously wholly Soviet-oriented Arab country, Iraq, toward the West, at first economically, as the better-endowed supplier of the wherewithal for a henceforth massively oil-financed economic development.

Similar inflections from the expected are apt to continue to

occur in both the most volatile issue and conflict areas and elsewhere. It is, therefore, more than normally useful to fix in time the
conception of any effort at analysis and evaluation. The most specific parts of the policy analysis and critique in what follows were
presented in their final form as a paper circulated and discussed at
a meeting of the Washington Center of Foreign Policy Research on
February 20, 1975—i.e., before the dramatic aggravation of the
military situation in Vietnam and the "suspension" of step-by-step
diplomacy in the Middle East escalated the criticism of Kissinger's
statecraft from issues of general conceptual approach (traditional
balance of power) and diplomatic style to policy substance and
results. In the following weeks I expanded and rearranged the
shorter paper, adding the more general or speculative observations
on statecraft and scholarship as well as the discussion of the
American-Soviet détente as the keystone of the conservative (or
Metternichian) design. The latter I did largely in response to objections suggesting that my original evaluation of Kissinger's statecraft in terms of the manipulative (or Bismarckian) model alone
did inadequate justice to the subject's real, conservative strategy. I
gratefully acknowledge the role of the fellow-members and the
guests of the Washington Center who forced me to rethink and
expand the basic structure of the essay, without burdening them
with any responsibility whatsoever for my views and arguments
regarding both specific and general points of policy, with many of
which they tend to disagree.

April 24, 1975

BEYOND KISSINGER:
WAYS OF CONSERVATIVE STATECRAFT

Studies in International Affairs Number 26

I. "ANTI-KISSINGER": PERSPECTIVES AND PREJUDICES

In his youth, in the intervals between playing the flute and dreaming enlightened despotism, the not yet great Frederick of Prussia wrote a book entitled *Anti-Machiavel*. It is one of the many "idealistic" critiques of the Florentine's wicked statecraft. The instant Frederick became king, he reached for *Anti-Machiavel* and grasped, instead, *The Prince*. In due course the career of conquest led for him to the cleansing passion play of the Seven Years' War, instigated, in large part, by the differently constituted passion of the Habsburg empress at whose expense Frederick would make Prussia viable as one of Europe's great powers. It was Maria Theresa's first minister, Count Kaunitz, who gave his name to the coalition arrayed against the conquering Prussian in the second of the Silesian wars in the mid-eighteenth century. The "diplomatic revolution" which produced that coalition was, more even than the Peace of Westphalia, the formative event of the truly modern European international system, even while being the most recondite of the background events figuring centrally in this treatise.

The treatise as a whole must not be read as the exact parallel to Frederick's; this is not an "idealistic" critique of Kissinger as the authentically Machiavellian statesman. If anything, the obverse is the case. What follows is a critique in the tradition of Machiavellian scholarship of what is taken to have been Kissinger's "idealism" in foreign policy of a special kind. The operative side of this peculiar idealism has been a prudential nursing of trends, with a minimum of interfering strategic action, on the assumption that the trends were, on balance, beneficial. Its doctrinal basis has been in an overstatement of phenomena such as "moral consensus" and "legitimacy" as independent from power and evenly complementary with it. The actual realities underlying the first are less elevated, and the needs and possibilities attaching to the second less universal, than Kissinger's philosophic emphases might suggest, however. Thus "moral consensus," applied to the nineteenth-century historical setting which Kissinger highlighted in his scholarly writings, is all too often but the high-sounding label for conservative reaction, for restraint on the uses of power based on the transiently and unevenly shared fear of the renewal in the future of past revolutions; and the disinterment of the value of "legitimacy" in the post-revolutionary setting was in effect but a matter of diplomatic lobbying—a way for either imparting (by Talleyrand, at Vienna) ideological dignity to a very specific diplomatic objective or for infusing (by Metternich, more generally) political stability and ideological sanctity into the previously negotiated postwar settlement. The end result was reminiscent more of sclerosis than of spontaneity. Moral consensus has been more truthfully described for our time as the "negative community of interests" (between the two superpowers, in relation to shared dangers from nuclear weaponry, extensible more recently to dangers from social upheavals). At the same time, concern with legitimacy has been largely premature for an international system that, while it did weather a major war-substitute in the form of the cold war, has merely begun to evolve toward structures of eventual stability. It could not, therefore, be meaningfully legitimized at this early stage either at all or by virtue of a moral consensus between the two powers that happened to be ahead of the global procession at this particular juncture.

The estimation of Kissinger's statecraft as "idealistic" in these terms is neither widely shared nor self-evident; prudential statecraft has increasingly, if falsely, preempted the full meaning of political "realism." It will take an entire little volume to make the patient reader see how much, if any, basis there is for the contention. But a caveat must be inserted at the outset: to tax Kissinger with philosophical "idealism" (albeit of the conservative vintage) is not the same as defending him automatically against imputations, right or wrong, of what can only be called vulgar Machiavellianism, in the form of a deceitful approach to politics. Essential Machiavellian statecraft—and, derivatively, scholarship—embodies a more elevated conception of political activity. This conception relates the term, instead, to the lucid acceptance of, and creative response to, the "necessities" implicit in the competitive rise and decline of political organisms by the morally self-sacrificing and strategically innovative servant of the Reason of State. The

Machiavellian statesman, consumed as he is by the passion for power *and* service, willingly incurs all attendant risks to his immortal soul (or whatever may be the current equivalent) without regard for either mundane acclaim in the present or posthumous approval in history.

As they surface, the themes in the treatise are carried along by the conviction that Kissinger's statecraft has not measured up to that kind of exalted standard. The critical analysis which results is thus sympathetic, in that it does not go outside the general framework of reference (classic statecraft) which is widely identified as being Kissinger's; and it is prejudiced in the just-mentioned evaluative sense. From the very beginning of Kissinger's official tenure, there was academic criticism of his supposed commitment to nineteenth-century, or balance-of-power, statecraft. The approach was decreed obsolete by scholars of standing; but Kissinger's mastery of the art was, both implicitly and explicitly, all the more affirmed. It is the basic argument here that the report of Kissinger's greatness as a traditional statesman was exaggerated at best and certainly premature, and that the basic premises behind the antitraditionalist criticism partook of the same debility. If one part of the critique has overstated Kissinger's mastery of ancient mysteries, the other has overdone the novelty of modern developments and dilemmas. Since the fashionable critique mistakes the practical range of international statecraft, it mistakenly calls off the classic "game" before all the players have retired to the cooling showers. After each testing or exciting period, the temptation grows strong to find refuge in whatever is the momentarily apposite variety of "economism" and, in some form, organizational "institutionalism." Since just before the French Revolution at the very least, periods of strategic-diplomatic détente or debilitation of the great powers (consequent upon spells of great exertions) have been occupied by more or less profound crises in social and economic structures that affect the next round of diplomatically or militarily enacted conflicts, even if they do not constitute their principal source. In our all-too-ready time, such détente-decay periods provide an irresistible invitation to the preachment of "diplomatic disarmament."

At its summits, where the giants of any denomination walk alone, diplomacy is the art of constellating and configurating forces, not of contriving formulae of policy compromises or bastions of universal peace and prosperity; the art of bending and aligning basic dispositions rather than bargaining over minutiae in implementing relaxation of political tensions or deploying peacetime military force. The second-mentioned efforts are essential and can be fascinating; but it is the first-mentioned ones that are preconditional and liable to be awe-inspiring. One may be wholly disposed to leave Kissinger's reputation as bargainer untouched on the assumption that the revealed record may one day confirm the rumored bases for it. One may be also prepared to agree that he was proven right as the conservative philosopher of interstate relations if, in two decades or so, events will have supplied an indisputable confirmation; if, that is, relations among the great powers have meanwhile continued unfolding toward ever-greater stability, and no major revolution in the intentions and objectives of any one of them required last-resort responses from relatively weakened residual capacities of the others. Pending such consummation, the principal critique of Kissinger's performance will be that he did not visibly try—or did not try effectively—by the traditional means of the highest order to globally consolidate and extend to the world's most troubled regions the opportunities offered by the dispositions of the two great Communist powers which he had found, ready and waiting, upon entering on his official responsibilities.

To substantiate the point will require replaying some, at least, of the key events and issues covered by Kissinger's tenure with the aid of hypothetical reasoning, even while assessing the constraints within which Kissinger admittedly had to operate. Hypothetical strategic reasoning of the diplomatic kind is not a widely favored type of mental effort in this country. More congenial to both material and intellectual American endowments is the utopian-fabian mix of great expectations to be approached gradually through organization and management. If this means organizing solutions to finite problems, it means also managing complex processes by way of their most tangible components. This bias governed the dominant academic criticism of Kissinger's statecraft until personality and style were brought in by politicians emboldened by Kissinger's (temporary?) loss of charisma. If a different kind of criticism is offered here at all, it is because the diplomatic-strategic mode of thinking is an aptitude which a political culture allows to atrophy only at the price of peril to the political power it is supposed to leaven and sustain. To say that such reasoning and the related implementing statecraft are no longer needed because the principal world problems are elsewhere—no longer in the equilibria of power but in the equations and equities of human well-being—is, first of all, a blow below the belt. It appeals to sentiment while taxing the strategic statesman (or thinker) with illustrating man's inhumanity to man. And it is a push at an open door: there is no limit to the desire to believe this because, difficult as the "material" problems are, they can still be approached with small steps at a time. Nor do they raise the kind of moral and political responsibilities which attach to the grand strokes of creative or manipulative diplomacy.

Subsequent pages illustrate the strategic mode of thinking in diplomatic statecraft. This is done without any pretense of providing the best possible demonstration of the method or offering the best possible substantive policies. On its most positive side, this treatise is a plea for an approach and not for a particular alignment of policy; it is an effort to keep aglow a special kind of ardor rather than to encompass the generality of the world's ills. The political philosophy and shrewd political insights of the founding fathers have not much more to teach in this area of intelligence than has the philosophy of Karl Marx; and it may not be possible to cull all the necessary directives from the philosophy and practice of the most controversial American secretary of state since Dean Rusk. It is a safe prediction that both this country and, if and when they awaken from the long sleep, the ancient civilizations of Europe and Japan will for some time yet need to count as "powers among powers." As for the United States alone, whether it is to be preeminent, paralyzed in deadlock, or declining will in large part depend—all the "projects interdependence" to the contrary notwithstanding—on the survival, in the recesses of the collective mind and at the heights of national policymaking, of the arts and crafts of a Bismarck, a Kaunitz, and even of the hero of Kissinger's own earlier years, Klemens von Metternich.

II. MACHIAVELLIAN SCHOLARSHIP: CONCEPTIONS AND CONSTRUCTS

In the person of Henry Kissinger the United States has acquired the first fresh experience since Woodrow Wilson of the academic scholar in a commanding position in international statecraft. Simultaneously, and contrarily to the Wilsonian era, the reentry of scholarship has coincided with a second major spell of the classic mode in American foreign policy, following Theodore Roosevelt's exercise in manipulative diplomacy in the flexible setting of several great powers. The two developments taken together amounted to a marriage of traditional international-relations scholarship with classic international statecraft. The event encourages speculation about the relationship between the two branches of activities concerned with international relations that may usefully precede the critical analysis of Kissinger's statecraft while reaching—as does the analysis, more extensively and descriptively—back to earlier periods and individuals who embody the classic approach in forms relatively unalloyed with forces and processes that have since complicated its exercise without superseding its utility.

I

It is left for later chapters to analyze and offer a critique of a particular statecraft. They will do so from a particular perspective and from the vantage point of a specific moment in time (January-March 1975). As a result, in the best of cases, the value of the analysis is in large part ephemeral; and it is contingent on the amount of more enduring "truth" it has discerned and expressed. With further passage of time the perspective is apt to change: the apparent failures of one day may still be the successes of another (and vice versa); and even the overall setting can undergo upheavals which reduce to the status of idiocy both insights and initiatives that appeared to be incisive at the time of their conception. What is true or right changes with time in a political universe that is infinitely complex and both continually and dialectically evolving. What has ceased to be true or right at one time can become so again from a yet longer temporal distance. The factual chaff, the tactical minutiae, is perishable; the presently far-fetched outlines of systems and strategies can actually emerge to unsuspected validity as reality evolves through action and counteraction, progress and regress, and as the mind discounts the clutter of circumstance which, all-absorbing in one instant, shrinks to its real significance—or insignificance—in the next instant.

To say so much is already to imply that critique must occur in a conceptual setting if it is to have an intellectual significance exceeding its immediate practical function: to keep discussion of policies going, to signal one's superior wisdom, or to show that the pen is mightier than the sword—or the secretaryship of state. It must be part of an at once disciplining and elevating construction. This is not the same as saying that criticism must be constructive in the commonsense meaning of directly helpful. But neither does it mean that, being an art form about an activity (statecraft) which itself is better understood as art than as exact science, critique is—or ought to be—an art for its own sake. If critique as part of a theoretical construction, or construct, does have an aesthetic dimension, that dimension consists less of literary elegance of expression and more of internal coherence or balance. Sympathetic exposition must be amended by significant criticism, the sweeping panorama by the revealing or salient detail, explicitness by allusiveness or even—when it best reflects the ambiguity of what is, and stimulates the reader's independent groping for its meaning—elusiveness. To be always precise and explicit in matters political is to be sometimes (or even oftentimes) inaccurate and misleading; the subtly formulated abstraction may be more descriptive than the blunt, positive affirmation.

Furthermore, the critique-oriented construct will usefully draw in considerations from outside the topic of immediate concern, be they historical or speculative. As it does so, the scholarly undertaking reaches beyond the aesthetic dimension to its more pertinent purpose: to instruct about statecraft in general as well as to enlighten about the works of an individual practitioner. In the process, the scholar sets up ideal and demanding standards which the practitioner cannot fully meet or satisfy, and against which the reviewed set of events and accomplishments can be projected without being more precisely measurable. The standards are derived from two principal sources. One is the romance of the great deeds of statecraft, performed by its peculiar heroes. Those statesmen are "great" who knew how to employ for fundamental creation the limited reach and superficial means of foreign policy. They knew when, where, and how to apply the accessible handles or levers to the individual and aggregate forces and energies which are beyond direct shaping and interference at their foundations. They knew, in other words, how to identify and then relate to the intended purpose the last and most accessible link in the endless chain of social causation. The other source of standards of judgment is the more general and anonymous process of politics in the system of states itself. It generates standards as it unfolds over time in both recurrent cycles and overall evolutionary progression, and as it registers the interplay of human will, situational compulsion, and changing material wants and means.

The two together—the great deeds and the gradual development —are the quarry from which to mine insights about an undertaking which is suspended between the sublime and the humdrum. The sublime inheres in the stakes, revolving as they do about the growth, the crises, and the decline of the framework of civilized life in organized polity. Were it not for this, there would be no valid reason for men's awe before the great builders and movers of states. In the best of cases, their work is subject to all the routine trivialities of the statesman's craft, except for the unique capacity to divine and to dare: divine when and how to act on key occasions, and dare act when action is called for. The sharp contrast between the two poles—the sublime and the trivial—is the source of a tension, one of several, which energizes the best in statecraft and which the "realistic" or "Machiavellian" scholar must strive to reproduce with his still more limited means.

What is the immediate significance of this for policy criticism? It is that a critique must occur within a positive construct or schema which directs attention to the setting in wider systems and strategy of the specific features which are unlikely to be readily overlooked in any event. The schema is apt to be more abstract than concrete; and its purpose is to afford perspective more than to facilitate prescription. It implies standards of evaluation while prompting substantive evaluative conclusions without dictating them. The purpose is not to produce or encourage detailed, shot-by-shot criticisms or to prescribe in detail specific alternative policies. Both are beyond the scholar's primary function. When overindulged in, they reduce the scholar to surrogate statesmanship without endowing him with the necessary tools and without charging him with corresponding responsibilities. If he is not supernaturally endowed with information, intuition, and practical or applied intelligence, the scholar who attempts to preempt the role of the statesman will only discredit himself in due course, and his calling; he will become, sooner or later, the academic knight of the sad countenance thrown off by the windmills of his own creation. A specific and detailed criticism, if it is retrospective, is apt to be in large part gratuitous "if everything were known"; too-particular policy suggestions, if prospective, are apt to isolate the tree from the forest—to "optimize" one issue to the detriment of the remainder.

The schema or construct employed in the forthcoming analysis is many-faceted. It consists of three sets of three elements each, and two pairs. The first triad is that of style, (diplomatic) *système*,[1] and (international) system. The three diplomatic systems that are reviewed are identified with historically prominent statesmen of the eighteenth and nineteenth centuries. The structure of the international system is dealt with as tripolar, encompassing the United States, the Soviet Union, and China as the major contemporary powers. In addition, two levels (of smaller and greater states) are viewed as bounded by two basic structures of power (multipolar equilibrium and one-power hegemony). The style-*système*-system triad encompasses one kind of range along a spectrum which extends from the formal to the material, from the specifically individual and even subjective to the cumulatively and collectively evolved and—consequently—largely objective. It thus reflects the basic characteristic of statecraft as an activity defined by the interplay of freedom and necessity, with choices narrowing as issues and contexts become more critical and affect actual "survival." A statesman or a policy élite is relatively freest to choose a style; the diplomatic system is comparatively more contingent for efficacy on its fit with an international system (in the sense of

---

[1] I follow the original usage of the term in diplomatic practice and literature and refer to a particular statesman's particular diplomatic strategy and preferred configuration.

power and conflict distribution), and the international system is, to a large extent, the matrix of situational compulsions whose existence the practicing statesman is able to deny with less impunity than may the voluntaristically inclined scholar.

Styles of conduct in general have their importance, and so has diplomatic style. It is a mistake, however, to single out style for emphasis as if it were independent of status and situation in the international system and flowed instead from a unique group culture or from .an original or imitative personal idiosyncracy. The idiosyncracy can be Metternich's or Kissinger's; the distinctive group culture be American versus European or, within the latter group, British versus French versus German, for instance. More than either culture or idiosyncracy, however, the more or less rationally implemented style of diplomatic action expresses the individual's or nation's situation or circumstance. The different propensities to bargaining, assertiveness, legalism, opportunism, restlessness, or absolutism (alternation between total war or total peace) express the relationship between goals and means, the margins of available international credit and national capital relative to the prevailing contingencies and crises. The American diplomatic style was of one kind in conditions characterized by America's pretentious impunity—or safe pretence—which ended only recently. It changed sharply and rapidly with the onset of the constraints implicit in continuous involvement in international politics—in the balancing of power against power as compared with scavenging on the power struggles of others. Some elusive characteristic biases and propensities may have residually survived in practice—thus "absolutism" (as defined above) and self-deception about goals and motives. These are, however, not distinctively American, and they are secondary to the impact of the operative diplomatic style, which reflects the present American situation in the international system more than it reflects an American culture rooted in an increasingly irrelevant past. Who would dispute that contemporary American statecraft is more in the style of a Castlereagh, for instance, than of a Cleveland; more in the style of a Richelieu than of a Theodore Roosevelt? Or who could argue that the diplomatic style of Weimar or Bonn Germany was that of Bismarckian or Wilhelminian or Hitlerian Germany?

And if there are similarities in the diplomatic styles of a Metternich and a Kissinger, they are questionably due to a common, Germanic, cultural background (apt to be very different in specifics in any event). Nor are they wholly due to Kissinger's intellectual assimilation or actual imitation of Metternich's lifestyle (exhibited in the first Nixon administration), his diplomatic style (surfacing mainly in the second term including the Ford presidency), or his pretended political philosophy. Kissinger's "Metternichian" style expresses also, and more significantly, his estimate of the position or situation of the United States, its relative power and will, in the existing political world. That estimate may be correct or not, may be profound or fasten on a transient collective mood; but it has been essentially rational and functional. The same is true for any possible parallels between the styles of Kissinger and Bismarck. In this case, the style is not conditioned by a bias to avoid risks in the face of massive or compact impediments to either self-assertion or breakthrough (as it is in the Kissinger-Metternich parallel). It is conditioned by a bias toward juggling both domestic and external factors in a universe that is fragmented (internally with respect to consensus and externally as regards multiplicity of policy centers and issues). And supposing that there is a Kissinger style synthetizing the Bismarckian and Metternichian style traits, expressed in tactical juggling as a means of avoiding the risk of too-daring strategies and in diplomatic activism as a safeguard against critique from missed opportunities, it would likewise reflect Kissinger's perception of his situation in the domestic and international environments at least as much as anything else.

It is easy to overindulge in the dissection of diplomatic styles in isolation from the diplomatist's situation, if only because both the effort and the results are highly captivating and supply relief from more austere forms of policy analysis. Any reservation about style points to the diplomatic system as the connecting link—the *trait d'union*—between the subjective or individual features and the objective or systemic facets. Style can be seen, even if wrongly, as a determinant of international behavior without systemic cause or constraint. No such view can be taken of the relation of a specific diplomatic system to the structure of the international system. A fanciful *système*, one out of keeping with the structure of power and conflicts, is of course possible to imagine; and it will be occasionally essayed as part of a desperate effort to restore a declining power—such as, typically, seventeenth- and eighteenth-century Spain—again to the forefront of powers, or else as part of an undertaking—such as Woodrow Wilson's—to place an ascendant power before its time ahead of all the other powers. Such a foreign-policy conception verging on conceit may last awhile. It will have a shadowy existence as long as it is sustained by either a compensating power surplus of the state itself or an upholding deadlock among other major states; as long as it enjoys the advantage of practical irrelevance or is to the temporary advantage of other and more relevant strategies. Sooner or later, however, the unrealistic *système* will be exposed to realities as they are, be tested by them, and fail to resist the consequences of its mis-fit with them.

The three diplomatic systems delineated later on in this essay were appropriate for the situation and the objectives for which they were conceived and applied. And, apart from their immediate function, they delimit the range of basic prototypes in a multi-power or balance-of-power situation. The range from Bismarck via Kaunitz to Metternich, while distorting chronological sequence historically, coincides with the always-present range encompassing an ascendant power, a relatively declining but still strong power, and a both relatively and absolutely declining weak power. In that sense the range encompasses the organic dimension of inter-state relations which vitally interplays with the balancing or mechanical one. The crucial significance of the interplay between the two dimensions for international politics cannot escape the notice of anyone who contemplates the careers of states and nations over a long period of time. By the same token, it tends to be ignored in analyses that focus on too narrow a segment and too short a time span and tend to see an "end of history" in climactic contemporary events—such as, in our time, America's ascent to world power or the resolution of the ideological and political East-West conflict.

Ordering representative diplomatic systems along the rise-decline continuum suggests two insights. One is that salient diplomatic systems will coincide with major turning points in the rise-decline dynamic of individual great powers and in the collective responses to that fluctuation. It is these, therefore, that deserve particular attention, rather than single dramatic events such as military engagements, peace conferences, or institutional innovations, which may only implement critical stages in ascent or descent. The other insight is that the statesman, even when dealing offensively or defensively with such fateful turning points, is largely confined to an essentially superficial and manipulative role externally and to corresponding measures and instruments. This may not appear to be true in all cases. A Richelieu may have won greatness, as the architect of French power, by virtue of his laborious restoration of domestic order even more than because he subsequently managed alliance politics in the last phase of the Thirty Years' War with a mastery that reestablished France as the again ascendant power. If so, the case would be an exception that confirms the rule, however. When a twentieth-century Frenchman tried to reenact Richelieu's dual achievement by starting with the domestic base, he failed by his own standard when the international setting proved resistant. Nor were Bismarck's internal preliminaries to the unification effort by Prussia, while essential for the military mobilization of national capability, equal in decisive importance to his international constellations. While Richelieu's internal task (to gain and hold the king's support in constraining the fractious nobles) was tactically difficult, moreover, it was inherently easy when compared with the issues raised by more complex or built-in social and economic forces and problems that will be typically involved in organic expansion or constriction of a political community. Thus the direct and traceable contribution of the Hohenzollern dynastic statecraft to the early rise of Prussia through internal management could not be replicated by comparably identifiable deliberate planning and performance in the more broadly based continuance of that growth in modern Germany. Similarly, even when the essential components of decline as a problem have been correctly analyzed by contemporaries—as was the case for declining Spain and, more recently, France—and intelligent and even masterful statesmen attempt a remedy, it has been beyond human resource to reverse the process with the resources of domestic statecraft, either alone or primarily.

The management of decline by internal statecraft is more difficult than is that of rise. It is decline, moreover, which has historically constituted the greater problem for international statecraft as well. Classic theory of the balance of power could indulge in appearances of equity by removing internal growth from among the legitimate incentives to reactive or repressive counterbalancing, even while being silent on the issue of internal shrinkage. In practice, the balancing mechanism must be brought into action to deal with the erosion of power at least as often as with the exuberance of surplus power. And likewise in practice, reactive statecraft will have both sufficient time and compelling occasion to step in when the internal growth, which is theoretically exempt, has expressed itself in external conduct affecting others in ways experienced as threatening; it will, just as predictably, respond to internal decline when it has become manifest in an external predicament which only others can attenuate. The challenge is then to configurate extraneous power in such a way as to counteract the vortex effect which a major power's abrupt sinking would have on the international system in its entirety. The elasticities of modern economies and the flexibilities of modern social dynamics may have modified and eased somewhat the problem of decline. But they have neither disposed of it in its material aspects nor basically moderated its aggravation by perceptual or psychological reactions.

The ambiguity of balance-of-power theory regarding most intimate internal developments reflects the weakness of formal or normative limits on international statecraft most of the time and its attempts at fair play some of the time. The actual incapacities of statecraft in the domestic arena express in turn the major material limitation of international statecraft which grows whenever internal factors do not respond readily to the needs of foreign policy or cannot be manipulated by foreign policy. Both Metternich and Bismarck tried to have an impact on their domestic scene: the first, haphazardly, with the aim of moving it closer to strength through orderly repose; the second, more persistently, by fragmenting political opposition and containing by social reform forces inimical to the traditional domestic order and, along with it, to the primacy of foreign policy. But the prime role and refuge from domestic inhibitions for both was in the international arena, as a field in which to strengthen one's hand and weaken the adverse pressures operative within. The internal standing of both—as well as that of the internally more immune Kaunitz—rested squarely on their mastery of the relations with other powers; if in the end they both fell over "revolutionary" internal issues, Metternich actually and Bismarck ostensibly, this corroborates the intractability of such issues more than it demonstrates an insufficiency peculiar to the compensatory foreign-policy recourse.

Nothing works for ever and in all circumstances. Nor is the prime role of international statecraft in adjusting the framework for comparatively more autonomous internal processes only a historical fact without current relevance. All major American presidents have instinctively gravitated to foreign affairs in search of identifiable accomplishment and in quest of both a lever on and an escape hatch from the complexities of internal problems. To take this course was thus not in our time the prerogative of an anachronistic traditionist such as France's Charles de Gaulle. The "primacy of domestic politics" as both doctrine and practice is the recourse, probably only temporary, of nations, such as contemporary West Germany, which labor under the sense of earlier abuse of the contrary principle and enjoy the political comforts of economic prosperity at the same time. More generally, domesticism will reign when a stalemate among powers momentarily paralyzes the international dynamic; or when a phase of interstate turmoil has temporarily yielded to détente as part of the repetitive cycle of crisis and subsidence which marks international relations over longer periods of time. By contrast, domesticism does not reliably hold sway when the domestic situation is in profound crisis, since only external resorts may then either help resolve the related intergroup conflicts or distract attention from them.

Quintessential international statecraft is thus a matter of divination: divination of the right constellation and the appropriate leverage for effecting and consolidating that constellation. The intuitive guess precedes in both logic and in time the effective manipulation of the forces in existence, and it is qualitatively different from a deliberate management of the elements of power to be nursed into being only gradually. The inescapable paradox is that this most superficial of tasks requires, for success, the most penetrating of insights and the most subtle of executions. The statesman, to be great, must first master and then implement the paradox; the international-relations scholar, to be realistic, must perceive the existence of the paradox in principle and then try to comprehend and expound the different forms assumed by its implementation. He must not, that is, turn to the tempting depths of sociological and related inquiries alone or even primarily, in implied contempt of transactions over against transformations. It just may be that he can, in the end, understand the sources of conduct and the dynamics of societies and economies no better than even a great statesman can shape and direct them.

Since the structure of the international system is the prime conditioning factor of the diplomatic system, its careful delineation is indispensable for evaluating that latter system's efficiency and fit. It is true that the rightness of a policy tends to be equated in casual criticism of international action with its visible success. However, the so-called realistic approach to international relations does not have the monopoly on the world's injustice to even magnificent failure. On the contrary, a sensitively applied academic extension of the Reason-of-State doctrine has, built into it, standards of appreciation keyed to technical excellence, to virtuosity in the art, which are independent of blatant success and immediate payoff. Like many other things, including loyalty and betrayal, success may be a question of dates and depths. Hence the ultimate rightness of the Kaunitzian reversal of diplomatic alignments despite its early drift toward final failure; and hence the questionable rightness of Metternich's conservative statecraft in different time perspectives, despite self-serving exaltation by Metternich himself and the exaggerated plaudits by some latter-day historians. Conversely, was Bismarck's complex diplomatic system of checks and balances ultimately wrong despite its initial success? Or was only style at fault, in its bias to forcible action, when it was perpetuated by both lesser and still-more-ambitious men? The question so put supplies its answer: the diplomatic system was wrong only if it is assumed that both its extension in scope and aims and its simultaneous simplification in alignment structure by Bismarck's successors were latent in the system from its inception: that is to say, if they were the unavoidable reaction to the system's procedural complexity (its counterpoising principle) and its substantive confinement (to mainly continental scope, failing to do justice to the widely postulated imperatives of the contemporary world political economy).

All three of the diplomatic systems were related to a comparable structure of international politics, comprising several major powers and key conflicts. Such a structure is the prerequisite of full-blown balance-of-power politics. Consequently, the fit or lack of fit between the international and the diplomatic systems was more precisely a function of the organic dimension: the way in which the originating statesman's power base as either rising or declining dovetailed with the rise-decline configuration of actual or potential allies and adversaries. The relevant trends involve both the material factor of usable power and the imponderable factor of basic dispositions: assertive (revisionist) or restrained (conservative), stable or volatile, intermittently or continually involved. An international system in an advanced stage of evolution is apt to encompass a wide range of mutually complementary powers and dispositions and to be sustained by the resulting facilities for the politics of equilibrium. Conversely, the classic-modern European system was beset by a structural difficulty which it never surmounted and over which it finally went down in ruins. This was the schism between the maritime power—Great Britain, with its narrow land base—and the big continental powers with maritime and colonial ambitions—following Spain, France, and still later, Germany. The schism conditioned and frustrated the Kaunitzian system most directly; it affected the Bismarckian system at first positively as a latent background factor and was brought to bear on it overtly and destructively when the growing naval and colonial ambitions of post-Bismarckian Germany revolutionized the Anglo-French-German triangle; and the cleavage affected the Metternichian system least directly and most propitiously by augmenting the tactical diplomatic options of an Austria that had renounced other than strictly local maritime and "colonial" ambitions.

The present situation in a comparatively "new" or "young" global international system has displayed a twofold structural impediment, which has impeded the literal or integral applicability of either of the three diplomatic systems. One, there has been at best only a tripolar or three-power structure; and two, the rise-and-decline status and related dispositions of the United States and of the two great Communist powers relative to the United States and to one another have been highly ambiguous and indeterminate. The superficial impression is clear enough as far as the United States itself is—or perceives itself as being—conservative in mood and either still rising relative to others or stabilized in material power. The two Communist powers appear to be unsatisfied with their present status, expanding in their absolute and relative material power, and thus potentially reassertive on a grand scale. This ambiguity impedes final commitments and stabilization almost as much as did the land-sea power cleavage historically. Sea power has remained important in limited politico-military contests and for strategic nuclear deterrence; and it continues to impinge on the issue of commerce and communications. But the structural dilemma posed for the balance of power by the land-sea power schism has been attenuated by postcolonial transformations in world economy, by the substitution of the nuclear for the naval ultimate weapon, and by changes in the role and utility of the oceans as the proximate stake. If nuclear military technology transcends differentiations of terrestrial space, the oceans are being assimilated to territory for economic purposes and are enlarging it in the process.

In the prevailing structural and organic conditions, both statecraft and scholarly analysis must keep their options open. The first must accomplish this by manipulating effectively, and the second, intellectually, alternative potential constellations as part of the enduringly valid "classic" strand, without final commitment to either of the so-called alternative futures. The statesman explores the *ad hoc* possibilities of deriving a specific or local advantage from particular configurations of weights and pressures by the powers on one another, even while he does all he can for the more "basic" or "constant" factors. The scholar with a commitment to the classic approach engages speculatively in the same kind of enterprise as a means to delineating a "maximalist" diplomatic solution to salient issues (of regional war and peace or global equilibrium). The maximum sets up a standard or framework for judgment of what is legitimately the more prudent or "minimalist" approach by the statesman most of the time. Moreover, ideally, the scholarly delineation is the means to demonstrate by implication not only theoretical possibilities but also practical impossibilities, by pushing the alignment variations (or institutional arrangements, etc.) to their extreme and logical limits. The exonerating supposition is that the scholarly *reductio ad absurdum* is either a valid critique or a valid instruction, and cannot avoid being at least one of the two if competently performed. It suggests either where the statesman could or should direct his efforts or, alternatively, where he ought to fear to tread because the risks and costs appear to be sufficiently serious "on paper" to bar experimenting along the same lines in the field. A deliberately explicit scheme—such as that employed in the later analysis—helps organize and discipline that which is inchoate and elusive, polarize that which will overlap and interpenetrate in fact, and circumscribe that which may extend actually into an ever-widening circle of relationships. It may over-schematize formally; but it will distort materially only when its purpose is not understood—which is possible—or if it is applied literally in the area of action—which is unlikely.

That which is true for the three-times-three part of the schema is likewise so for its two-times-two segment. The first pair differenti-ates the great-power level and the smaller-power level. This is a commonplace enough distinction. But it bears being made firmly explicit and applied systematically in an analysis which concen-trates on relations among the great powers in particular. Choosing the great-power focus is natural for an analysis of statecraft in general which stresses diplomacy in a broad meaning of the term. Approaches with a less classic orientation can profitably affirm the growing importance of differently endowed smaller states and may even claim for them an unprecedented importance. Such analyses tend to discount the fact that small states were important before, even more important than they are today. They were so on the basis of either disproportionate financial strength, due to a fortui-tous commercial advantage, or of special assets, due to geography or specific military-technological endowments. Any single advan-tage did wonders in the age before the capacity to mobilize a huge population and exploit a vast territorial base temporarily pre-empted all there was to effective power. Even while important, however, the lesser states (a Savoy or the Swiss cantons or a Genoa or even Venice) did not, or not for long, prevail over and against the authentic great powers of the day. Analyses focusing on smaller states today have their validity, when they deal with forms of political processes different from those properly sub-sumed under the label "high policy": a policy—or diplomatic strategy—which sets the configurational framework for political or economic integration and interdependent or competitive functional relations. Such analyses go too far if they postulate the irrelevance of "high policy"; they can do so only in a foreshortened perspec-tive confined to isolated events, or by mistaking ideologically in-spired anticipation for analysis of what is.

In a classic worldview the great powers still call the shots. If, indeed, statecraft unfolds on the surface of things, the "power" which critically matters is the complete or composite power encompassing in a coherent aggregation both economic, military, and political factors or elements—those inherent in an individual state and those deriving from its situation in the systemic network. This is the only power which can be directly and effectively projected into diplomatic constellations with stable effects. Individual small states may well be onesidedly powerful (e.g., in a particular economic sector); and they will be more often negatively powerful (i.e., by virtue of their capacity to withhold assets or obstruct or derange relations among other powers). They are, then, important when their peculiar kind of power affects and inflects the relations of the great powers among themselves—when the great powers respond to the actual or potential impact of the lesser states on their own positions relative to one another, rather than reacting directly to the lesser powers. Moreover, the more limited is the leverage which great powers are able to exert directly and forcibly over small states, the more will they be anxious to affect the latter by way of the leverage they can exert over one another in the individually more reliably rational and mutually more responsive universe of inter-great-power relations. These are relations of settled states with relatively enduring and stable stakes in both specific issues and ongoing and cumulative relationships; of states that habitually react to pressures implicit in constellations which can outflank physically or isolate politically and can either elevate or depress formal status.

Such dangers and rewards are less significant among the lesser powers as long as they can draw on the greater ones to compensate for unequal weaknesses and strengths. This general premise warrants emphasis on the triangular interplay among the great powers, and the interplay between these and the small powers, as being critical for the development of regional balance-of-power systems in the Third World and for the diplomacy of peacemaking in the Middle East and Southeast Asia. A related emphasis is on the role of supplemental leverages to be derived from a thus expanded field of forces. The apparent opposite of such a manipulative approach is either surrender to a spontaneous socio-political process or a solicitous mediation appealing to the "real" interests and the "reasonable" dispositions of the contending parties in a diplomatically relaxed and militarily defused local and global environment. In actuality, however, the processes of both spontaneous evolution and of reasonable accommodation will unfold in the best of cases only superficially in separation from coercive or other inducements. They, too, will depend for effect on the interplay of pressure and counter-pressure; threat and promise; a dismal scenario versus a still more dismal one; and confrontation versus concert.

It would be a mistake to place confrontation and concert side by side as alternative approaches. So to place them is valid only as a device for sharpening the contrast between the two extremes and differentiating both from the intermediate gray area of limited cooperation and limited competition. In the real world, limited cooperation and competition occur against the backdrop of the more pronounced archetypes, as functions of the desire of parties to avoid more far-reaching concert or conflict while keeping both in reserve as a usable fall-back position and thus, in effect, a leverage. Moreover, a confrontation of varying intensity as a fact or imminent possibility will be commonly necessary to initially secure concert—or, more precisely, to secure adhesion to the costs of concerted action as well as its benefits by the more reluctant of the parties. Thus, for example, it may be necessary in due course to impose the concert format on the Soviet Union by recreating a confrontational situation before a superpower concert can "impose" a settlement on the lesser parties to the conflict in the Middle East. It would be easier to overcome any Soviet reluctance to put an end to the neither-war-nor-peace situation in the area if the Soviets could believe that the disappearance of the Arab-Israeli conflict would tend to surface other regional conflicts as a basis for their continuing influence. Even to hazard such a guess requires supplementing the two-level structural analysis (including great and small powers) with two-step strategic analysis. Such an analysis includes in reasoning the likely ulterior consequence of the first or immediate consequence in any process set off by an act of policy, while guessing whether the ulterior consequence will extend or reactively contain the immediate one.

Smaller states react upward to the greater powers more significantly than they do to one another horizontally, and the great powers interact horizontally rather than reacting downward to the lesser powers. This is the crux of the two-level interplay. The horizontal great-power interplay is, in turn, bounded by equilibrium among wholly equal states on one side and hegemony of one state or empire on the other side. Contrasting these extremes sidesteps the definitional and conceptual quibbles concerning the balance-of-power mechanism or principle, its theoretical validity in general, and its present applicability in particular.[2] The contrast delimits, however, one more, and not the least important, range. In the critical middle zone of this range spread degrees of superiority (or leadership) and inferiority (or need for adaptation) of the states interacting for equilibrium as a condition—or around equilibrium as a norm. Such interactions characterize a political oligopoly system of a few comparable, but not necessarily quite equally endowed, great powers. One of them may be the leader in the equilibrium interplay by virtue of its superior capacity for influencing the general tone and rules as well as exercising specific initiatives; but, with this qualification, all of the participant great powers will co-determine the degree of the possible mobility in pursuing stable and finite goals while eschewing both stultifying deadlock *and* excessive volatility. The range is a critical one for later discussion in that it delimits the boundaries of choice between an unqualified U.S. preponderance and a literal parity or equality, and suggests a practical alternative to either. It also points to the perennial phenomenon of a dynamic evolution and potential deterioration along the spectrum. In retrospect, the Nixon-Kissinger statecraft will score high or low depending on whether it effectively converted residual U.S. assets into an equilibrium leadership in relations with the Communist powers inferior in material capabilities and the variety of diplomatic options, or else was merely keyed to conspicuous diplomatic coups in exchange for uncompensated concessions.

The distinction between equilibrium and hegemony is likewise crucial for regional orders or systems of lesser states, as regards both long-term "structures of peace" and short-term pacification strategies. A peaceful stabilization is more likely to rest on either inter-party stalemate or one-party supremacy than on any special sophistication in bargaining or individual adjustments. Moreover,

---

[2] I examined those issues in *States in Evolution: Changing Societies and Traditional Systems in World Politics* (Baltimore: The Johns Hopkins University Press, 1973), pp. 152–66.

the question *cui bono*: To whose particular advantage? will arise both regionally and globally also with respect to transnational economic and other processes of interdependence. It will arise regardless of the hypothetical general benefit that might be held to result from them for the good of all. Such processes and relationships may one day become the sources of new international politics; so far they have been the most recent stakes of old international politics. As long as this is the case, both the further development of interdependence and the distribution of resulting benefits (and costs) will depend in large part on the infrastructure made up of the "composite" power of the major nations in particular. This infrastructure can crystallize only along the equilibrium-hegemony continuum; and both the new power assets and the new factors which are allegedly extraneous to "power" feed into evolving structures of conventionally constituted power and can be either sustained by those structures or be subverted by them.

An equilibrium situation is, on the face of it, preferable to one-power hegemony as the guarantor of rough equity in the distribution of assets and avoidance of injuries, inasmuch as mutual inhibition of drives and ambitions is a less precarious basis than is subjective good will. In actuality, however, integral equipoise, in which an "internationally minded" power does not exert leadership in defining the terms of different kinds of trades, can reinforce any existing tendency of contending great and small powers to adopt a mercantilistic (or beggar-thy-neighbor) approach to political economy. It will do so whenever, contrary to a certain theory, economic forces are not liberated from politico-military factors that had been neutralized by way of equilibrium interplays or any other way. Much depends on the size of the individual units and their consequent capacity to evolve viable self-contained politico-economic ensembles; and even more depends on the actual relations and dispositions of the major states. Thus, as they interact and influence one another over traditional stakes with both conventional and revolutionary means, the three great powers—and, if and when they move toward greater self-assertion internationally, Japan and Germany also—can either encourage or impede the perversion of interdependence into exploitation by small as well as great powers. At least two of the great powers can stand together in opposition to the one which incites the smaller states to "abuse" of their economic (e.g., raw-material) assets; or all three can vie over which can utilize the new leverage in international politics most effectively against the others. Which turn events take is not an automatic function of either socio-political ideology, comparative material endowments and needs of the different powers, or even the "inner logic" of economic (or any other) interdependence. It depends also on the price tag which one or the other great power can and will attach to undesired dispositions of both great and small states. The price can be in values qualitatively identical with those involved in the "new" network of interdependence—and can entail tests of relative economic strength most probably—or it can be defined supplementarily in traditional terms of more or less forcible and direct inducement. Especially coercive inducement will not be facilitated by integral equilibrium tantamount to deadlock. Nor would deadlock among actually "equal" great powers facilitate intervention for any other purpose. Intervention will, however, continue being an occasionally necessary moderating or ordering influence in lesser-power areas on local issues having little or nothing to do with the "new" international politics of transnational interdependence. It will be such even if officious and ubiquitous interference by great powers for selfish advantage or instant regional "peace" (i.e., cease-fire) has been sufficiently relaxed to permit the evolution of such areas toward relatively autonomous regional balance-of-power systems of their own by the only known means: competition and conflict.

Thus, it may be useful to push "reality" forward to its logical implications in areas of inquiry focusing on diplomatic systems and configurations. But there is also utility in restraint on inquiry. Reasoning or speculation ought not to go too far and too fast ahead of actualities in affirming novelties in international politics without a last backward look at the formative impact of traditionally defined structures and classic systems of diplomatic action on problems and processes that have been so far defined only conceptually, if at all.

II

Whatever the statecraft of a power like the United States may be committed to—regional peace or order through integration or balance-of-power systems; American world hegemony, or equilibrium leadership, or just equilibrium membership on the basis of all-round parity; national independence or transnational interdependence in critical material sectors—a major and continuing instrument for implementing the commitment will be diplomacy. Moreover, that diplomacy will be more or less directly and explicitly related to the uses of power in general and of force in particular. The question which will be implicitly raised in discussing Kissinger's statecraft is: What kind of diplomacy?[3]

On the plane of policies, the pertinent critical distinction is between routine diplomacy and creative diplomacy. Routine diplomacy smooths and implements established relations with the aid of only marginal adjustments. Its most constructive performance is in evolving formulas of mutually acceptable compromises which permit the existing configuration to endure and avoid thus the risks and convulsions of radical change. Conversely, creative diplomacy rearranges the setting within which negotiations for compromise occur. It does so by means of basic choices which are logically anterior to negotiations even when attended or implemented by such negotiations. The supreme expression of creative diplomacy is the "diplomatic revolution": a fundamental recasting or reversal of existing alignments which automatically marks a major stage (and a rare turning point) in the evolution of an international system. Revolutionizing diplomacy is not, therefore, to be confused with revolutionary diplomacy or statecraft attending a drive for boundless expansion externally or a fundamental socio-political reordering domestically. Creative diplomacy can be either of-

---

[3] Still more implicitly posed is the question of the distinction or relationship, if any, between diplomatic strategy (or *système*) and what Kissinger stressed in his academic writings under the term "doctrine"; between any such doctrine and a design; and, consequently, between strategy and design. It may or may not be correct to assume that Kissinger's doctrine meant either military doctrine in a narrow sense of the term (e.g., one governing the use of tactical nuclear weapons in an otherwise conventional warfare) or, in the broadest sense, a general philosophic attitude to international politics (e.g., the replacement of pragmatic responsiveness to events and adversaries by initiatives informed by a broad purpose, such as appeasement in depth following the exertions of the cold war and America's brush with tragedy over Vietnam). Our purpose is, however, even less to offer an exegesis of Kissinger's writings than it is to provide a detailed analysis of his style or substantive policies.

fensive or defensive in strategic purpose; and the transformation sought may be for repose as well as for major or continuing change. Bismarck's diplomacy was first offensive and then, after 1871, defensive; the diplomacy of Kaunitz (and of his French counterparts) compounded an offensive thrust with essentially defensive purposes; and Metternich's diplomatic choices were altogether defensive even when designed to facilitate localized offensive interventions. Metternich's statecraft, moreover, while experimenting with all of Austria's past alignment formulas, did not entail a major new alignment; it was revolutionary mainly in the commitment to great-power concert as a new institutional form or forum for alliance politics.

Whether offensive or defensive, a diplomacy that is creative to the point of revolutionizing the international system is in effect when a new, or just a different, conflict—or a new hierarchy of conflicts—is chosen to determine high policy in the sense of key alignments and dominant diplomatic strategy. In that sense it represents an exercise of freedom even while the existing configuration of acute and latent conflicts which the diplomacy converts into constellations circumscribes that freedom. The element of necessity grows as the range of practically possible effective choices narrows, and with it the scope for truly original or creative diplomacy. Thus when Kaunitz (in collusion with French opponents of the old *système* of Franco-Prussian alliance against the Habsburg House of Austria) undertook to induce French diplomacy to reverse its traditional alliance (and, in the process, turn to its "historical enemy"), he had two kinds of conflicts to work with and upon. France's conflict with Britain was overt and acute, involving as it did both immediate specific stakes (colonies) and general stakes (predominance in the European balance of power by virtue of mastery over world trade and maritime routes). This conflict could be pursued in alliance with either Prussia or Austria on the European continent, depending on which was more effective militarily and more likely to tie down British and release French resources for the decisive maritime-colonial arena. France's conflict with Prussia was, by contrast, sporadically acute only on the level of personal animosities and ambitions. Kaunitz's revolutionary diplomacy had, therefore, to surface—or make operational—the long-term or latent systemic conflict of France with Prussia (with

26

some help from the Prussian king's tactical miscalculations) and merge it with the more generally recognized disutility of continuing Franco-Austrian enmity. That is to say, Kaunitz had to first perceive and then effectively represent Prussia as France's principal long-term rival on the continent, as the ascendant German power which, if allowed to grow, would impede both the French political policy of influence in adjoining (western or Rhenish) parts of Germany and French anti-British military strategies in Germany's north and northwest. Similarly, the diplomacy of Bismarck had first to discern and then to exploit not only the acute estrangement of Russia from Austria, which could be turned into Russia's backing of Prussia, but also and more uniquely the latent new distance between France and Austria on grounds of nationality. It was that distance which gave Prussia the altogether critical assurance against simultaneous Franco-Austrian action on two fronts in one decisive military conflict.

Creative diplomacy rearranged the givens of the European balance of power within which routine diplomacy could again proceed with its appointed daily tasks. In the process, the higher form of diplomacy depended in both instances on manipulating both visible and latent conflicts, while balancing or re-balancing weights through new alignments conforming with perceivable but not generally perceived organic trends which involved both the traditional rise-and-fall dynamic and internal transformations attendant on the emergence of novel factors such as nationalistic sentiment. The contemporary equivalent of nationalism as a factor extraneous to the more constant elements in reason-of-state calculations has been ideology. It is, therefore, important for modern "classic" statecraft to properly guess at the extent and kind of ideological influences in the relations with as well as between the Communist great powers—and to foster a continuing atrophy of ideology by way of a more-than-usually-risk-taking diplomacy. This may mean assuming the risk of acting as if the Communist great power in question were more conventional in its goals (if not means) than it actually was in the particular instance. Or it may mean assuming the risks that are implicit in confronting such a power with maximum constraints on actions suspect of ideological motivation (or revolutionary implementation). In differing fashions and degrees, both approaches will aim to promote ideological erosion by creating either the occasion or an outright necessity for the carrier of a revolutionary ideology to deal with besetting "reality" in pragmatically effective ways.

Considerations involving the stateman's attitude to risk illuminate the difference between routine and creative diplomacy more than does any other single factor. The risk in question is not confined to the risk of war. As a general category, risk reflects the area of freedom in international relations, inasmuch as risk is meaningful only where there is a real choice between alternatives and, consequently, responsibility for the right or wrong choice. Where no choice exists, and complete necessity rules, it is meaningless to weigh the risks involved in a compulsion. The only choice left is one between the attitude of pathetic resignation to the inevitable and the attitude of heroic if unavailing (and thus tragic) revolt against it. From the viewpoint of the responsible statesman, the operationally significant risk of an action grows with the extent to which a consequence can be directly and unquestionably traced or assigned to such prior action. The consequence may be war; but it can also be only a setback or a different form of catastrophe. It is well known that Bismarck "doctored" the so-called Ems telegram, in which the Emperor described—without, in the original text, denouncing—a personal *démarche* by the French ambassador. The risk Bismarck took in changing the text for publication was that of unleashing war with France and of thus engendering the possibility of defeat for Prussia. While he favored war, defeat would have undone the previous success over Austria and terminated Prussia's role as unifier of Germany. The link between the revision of the telegram and the reversal of the Austro-Prussian balance in Germany back to Austria's advantage would have been direct and irrefutable. By contrast, for Metternich to choose alliance with a Bonapartist France (after Napoleon's abdication) over the opposition of Russia and Britain (favoring a Bourbon restoration) would not have entailed the immediate and certain risk of war. But the choice, if successfully implemented, would have disrupted the concert of the powers victorious over Napoleon; and, if frustrated, it would have sharply reduced Austrian influence in the concert of these powers. The gamble was adjudged not worth taking; the risks were too great from the viewpoint of a cautious diplomacy—although the immediate gain would have been even greater if the gamble had succeeded. Vienna would have been the effective center of European diplomacy for some time longer, rather than being merely the seat of a congress dominated by Castlereagh of Britain and Alexander of Russia and manipulated to a point by Talleyrand as the representative of Bourbon France.

More than once, the discussion that follows equates the style of Metternich and Kissinger in terms of aversion to risk and emphasizes the need for risk-taking in any effort to narrow a gap between diplomatic and international systems. It considers mainly risk inherent in traceable responsibility for failure, and it implicitly plays down the risk of a major nuclear conflict between the superpowers. But again, a risk of war can be involved, too. In the Middle East, for instance, had Kissinger eschewed the military disengagement of local belligerents in the October war of 1973 where it was apparently feasible as well as "necessary," and had he intensified instead the confrontation with the Soviet Union to the point where concert about political settlement appeared to be the only available alternative to converting confrontation into a directly or indirectly warlike conflict between the superpowers, his acts of commission and omission would have been directly traceable, and some form of "war" might have ensued or escalated, too. Conversely, if the United States had adopted, after military disengagement, a policy of conceding a circumscribed Hanoi supremacy in Vietnam or Indochina (involving a coalition government in South Vietnam), conjointly with an active manipulation of the triangular diplomacy (involving the contention between the two Communist great powers), it would have incurred no additional risk of renewed American participation in the Indochina war—additional, that is, to any existing feeling of obligation to demonstratively punish a ruthless seizure of total power in order to save American face. The policy entailed, however, the risk of a speedy Communist takeover in South Vietnam, directly traceable to the hegemonial peace strategy. The actually adopted contrary policy of continuing American aid to Saigon for resistance to Hanoi's hegemony was liable to protract the process of clarification and thus to shift immediate responsibility for an ultimate failure away from any one American policy-maker or executive policy. The cost incurred by the protracting strategy would be only in the hypothetical area of the possible positive consequences that the immediate risk-taking political settlement might have engendered for South Vietnam itself, the Hanoi-Washington relations, and America's relations with either or both of the Communist great powers.

It is in terms of this kind of distinction and reasoning that Kissinger's approach could be described as timid—i.e., devoted to a course of conduct which is safe in the short run from leading to an identifiable catastrophe. It is an extra bonus if the approach and related style are also satisfying for the statesman by permitting short-term successes none the less. And it is only an additional, and inherently disputable, confirmation of the presumption of timidity if the preferred conduct also includes a seeming preference for occasional strong language over against sustained hazardous action (for instance, in the Middle Eastern oil crisis or in relations with the European allies). The tendency of a statecraft intent on avoiding traceable responsibility to opt for lesser-risk alternatives reinforces the necessitarian bias that permeates international politics at the level of crisis. Thus, taking risks as part of a disarmament—or arms-control—strategy is the counterpart of a diplomatic strategy inclined to take the risk of war. The difficulty in realizing a major breakthrough in "disarmament" is due, first of all, to the competitive security dilemma of states. But the difficulty is aggravated by the decisional dilemma of the statesman, who will weigh the potential benefits of a major agreement or concession against the fact that any subsequent catastrophe would be more readily and directly traceable or attributable to the concession than to prior non-agreement due to the refusal to make such a concession. Many have argued that Kissinger took unwarranted risks in connection with SALT I and II. The risk-taking propensity that might be deduced from this is, however, discounted by the fact that nuclear-strategic equations are highly hypothetical, and the adverse effect of any present misjudgment is apt to be long-delayed; these attenuating circumstances will operate in favor of "risky" concessions when more pressing and immediate conventional issues—such as sustaining the political détente process with the aid of transactions in a relatively malleable symbolic area—are significantly at stake and have immediate priority.

At the back of the relationship between statecraft and risk in practice is the philosophic issue of the relation of diplomacy to war and peace. It highlights once again the difference between routine and revolutionizing, creative diplomacy. It has become common-place to identify diplomacy with the *preservation* of peace. The identification is strong also in the self-perception and post-retire-ment writings of the professional practitioners of routine diplo-macy. Its remote historical reason may be in a salient—though not the original—function of diplomacy in the classic period: the *negotiation* of peace terms (while war continued) and their ratifi-cation in a peace congress (when the war was ended or was about to end). The more proximate institutional reason is that the con-ceptual origination and primary execution of anything that is or purports to be more than routine diplomacy will automatically gravitate to a plane above that of the professional diplomatic class and will arouse its resentment on these grounds alone. The attitude is not confined to the war-peace issue. If a Louis XV had to use the "king's secret"—i.e., a parallel network of diplomatic agents—for effecting the diplomatic revolution, the more recent profes-sionals at the Quai d'Orsay (the French Foreign Ministry) were equally antagonistic to the efforts of a de Gaulle to recast relations with the Communist great powers in deviation from Atlantic or-thodoxy; and the hard core of State Department professionals were not particularly happy with the Nixon-Kissinger personal diplo-macy when it sidestepped the routinely established relations with America's allies for a similar objective. In other instances, the war-peace issue is directly involved. Thus the Wilhelmstrasse—mean-ing the German professional diplomatic establishment—was in the main opposed to Hitler's risk-taking diplomacy and matched the commitment of its French professional counterparts to peace. An apparent deviation from type in the 1930s was the anti-appease-ment slant of the dominant viewpoint in the British Foreign Office. Here the countervailing influence was, however, the older and more specific institutional tradition of hostility to Germany and support for the balance of power. Moreover, the "appeasement" policy joined the issues of peace and war on the one hand and of routine versus creative diplomacy on the other in an unorthodox manner. It was the peace-oriented appeasement strategy that was "revolutionary" insofar as it postulated a new *pattern* of the balance of power globally as compared with the traditional *proce-dures* of the balance of power intrinsic to historically routinized British statecraft vis-à-vis the continent of Europe.

More typically, the creative branch of diplomacy is not committed to peace for its own sake and in the short run. It is instead committed to positioning the state in such a way as to "optimize" its security and status with the least possible material exertion or forfeiture of political prestige. This involves, but is not confined to, consideration of the costs incurred in war. And it may require positioning the state for war, so as to conduct war with the greatest possible chance of success or to avoid it (by means of "deterrence") with greatest possible profit—i.e., while achieving at smallest possible material cost at least some of the positive results of a successfully concluded military conflict. Bismarck's diplomacy was preparatory to wars in its first phase, which led up to German unification; so was the Kaunitzian, prior to the Seven Years' War. Bismarck's second-stage diplomacy was aimed at preventing a war on two fronts while exhibiting a continuing readiness for war at the cost of "war scares" in support of a diplomatic preeminence exploiting the more immediately conflict-prone postures of the other powers. More recently, the American diplomacy of the Cuban missile crisis and of the military disengagement from Indochina depended critically on a manifested readiness for military engagement with one or both of the Communist powers. There is, of course, no negotiation for peace or any other object without an overt or covert confrontation of wills to be ultimately tested by the comparative readiness to contemplate and incur the consequences of the negotiations failing. This is the essence of bargaining in any arena; only the specific nature of failure and of its consequences differ from one arena to another. In the international domain, the threat or actual use of force of some kind is, therefore, a functionally required and ethically neutral instrument of diplomacy, a lever which is qualitatively on a par with economic pressures or interference in domestic affairs. It entails risks and consequences which are no greater, even if they are differently timed, than are the risks implicit in risk-avoiding drift.

Avoiding the use of force in the interest of saving lives is a valid humanitarian, but not a valid political, criterion for action. The political perspective is, or ought to be, both larger and longer. The problems involved have been increasingly critical for lower-level disorders, as use of force was paralyzed on the nuclear plane and inhibited on the higher levels of the conventional plane. An example may be derived from the so-called Pueblo case. The U.S. government refused to sacrifice (American) lives in staging a forcible response to what it characterized as piracy on the high seas. This was followed by the extension and growth of "piracy" both in the air (highjacking) and on land (abduction of foreign diplomatic personnel by urban guerrillas). In due course, the latter also supplied something of a test case for the relative merits of the humanitarian and the political response. The longer and larger view was seemingly justified when the wave of abductions appeared to subside only after some professional servants of peace, subjected to terrorism, were actually sacrificed to force by governments unwilling to continue being held up for ransom.

The commitment of the professional career diplomatist to peace against force has been matched by the elected officials of industrialized democracies in their public pronouncements and, increasingly, their policies as well. A tendency, spreading from the democracies in Western Europe to the United States, has been to confront the risks of conflict abroad by other than incremental decisions only or mainly when to avoid such risks would create yet greater and more immediate risks for political tenure internally. One such recent case was John Kennedy's dilemma in the Cuban missile crisis in the face of Republican disclosures and agitation. It is, however, more common for the basic desire to avoid traceable historical responsibility to be reinforced by the absence of an instant domestic penalty for avoiding the equivalent of moral heroism in foreign-policy action. Scholarship follows in the footsteps of the professional diplomat and the popular politician when it places the avoidance or resolution of conflict at the very top of its intellectual priorities and its research agenda. In so doing, it responds admittedly to salient technological (i.e., nuclear) facts and, impliedly, to prevalent popular (consumption-oriented) moods. But it also seriously distorts its optic on the phenomenon of international relations which it professes to study. This has been true especially for the approach to social and political events which prides itself on probing beyond the formal institutional facade to sources and patterns of behavior. In his attitude to conflict, the "behavioral" scientist has been a brother under the skin to the most formalistic professional diplomat, however. Whereas the routine diplomat resents the occasional revolutionizing statesman who pushes him aside, the methodologically or otherwise "revolutionary" scholar is typically inspired by an ideological resentment of the state as such and, by derivation, of organized power. The resentment is no less ideological for being concealed behind an elaborate screen of abstractions and vindicated by criteria that deny the theoretical utility of older concepts associated with the uncongenial phenomena. Far from being value-free, the compulsively peace-oriented approach is no more scientific than is that of the ideologue glorifying war and violence as such, in terms of their aesthetic or psychic worth, without reference to either objective conditions or rational objectives. Classic statecraft, with its dispassionate, instrumental approach to force, occupies the middle ground, which is appropriate also for effective and, indeed, scientific international-relations scholarship. There is no assurance of easy consensus even then. Thus a critic may—and an unfriendly critic will—detect a functionally unnecessary predilection for the forcible method in Bismarck's diplomacy, while an observer reacting to established perceptions will see a moderate-to-strong component of the instrumental approach to force in the international statecraft of Hitler.

So much for the outlook within which an evaluation of Kissinger's performance will be attempted. The ideal type of the risk-taking and system-revolutionizing statesman is no more than it pretends to be: one possible abstraction from historical realities both over time and contemporaneous. The implied criteria may be wrong in the sense that the ideal performance could either not be realized at all or could be attempted only at a risk which it would be irrational to entertain in prevailing circumstances. If a model were used that abstracted a different conception of the international system and statecraft and a differing reading of related historical events, perhaps those implicit in Kissinger's own writings, the assessment of Kissinger's performance would be different and might be higher. It might be much lower if the construct systematized the premises of transnational politics and world community.

The value of any more-or-less explicit construct or model is that it permits examination of the premises from which the critique proceeds. Moreover, it pits the skill and the authority of the critic more fairly against those of the object: the critic commits himself to a positive preference and even to a positive (if only intellectual) performance on his part before proceeding to negate, if negate he will or must. In exhibiting his entitlement to the critical role, he is free to employ any instrument at his disposal if the scales are to be balanced also in his favor relative to the practitioner. The display of historical knowledge, imperfect as it may be, expressed in the use of analogies, is as legitimate for the critic as it is for the practitioner when commending a policy (witness Bismarck's evocation of the "Kaunitzian coalition" for the edification of the Kaiser). The scholar may be more dependent on it, since the range of his instruments is still narrower than is the statesman's.

III

The issue of scholarly knowledge and entitlement raises the wider question of the relationship between international statecraft and scholarship. One form of examination is ruled out here: a textual explication of Kissinger's scholarly writings and the contrasting of these with Kissinger's doings on such specific issues as interallied diplomacy. Both the perspective and the functions of the scholar and the statesman are sufficiently different to entitle the scholar-become-statesman to turn his coat figuratively as well as to exchange it for one more accomplished sartorially. The real question is whether, and if so, how, the scholar related his academically evolved intellectual processes to the stringencies of practice in general.

There seem to be two basic responses to the problem: one may be called anti-conceptualist, the other, utopian. When adopting the first response, the previously theoretical academic writer casts aside his conceptual apparatus in order to be free to express his previously stifled drives in case-by-case "pragmatic" managing of issues and bargaining over issues. This solution may express the ex-academic's recognition that, upon closer inspection, his intellectual baggage did not include serviceable concepts and strategic ideas going beyond vague and general doctrines; or he may have insufficient confidence in the practical utility of strategic concepts and ideas derived from ratiocination rather than from action and experience. The other, utopian response will consist in an effort to apply academically derived concepts to international politics literally or mechanically. This solution may express a basic diffidence of the scholar as to his capacity to survive in the jungle of practice unless he has radically changed the modes and the rules of the game; or it may simultaneously express a deep-seated reformist or chiliastic commitment to converting the city of man into the city of god by act of intellect married to power and will. Among recent American scholars-turned-statesmen in international politics, Woodrow Wilson is closer to the latter type; Kissinger has been on balance the most recent and conspicuous representative of the lately more frequent and numerous first type. Thus also, in the European past, the "professors" formulating the strategies for German unification in 1848 were the intellectual utopians in foreign policy. In contrast to them, Bismarck was the conceptual statesman with no background in scholarship and no use for scholars in politics. Metternich fancied himself the philosophic statesman *par excellence*, while Kaunitz, in the best rationalistic manner of the Enlightenment, believed in the possibility of reducing foreign policy to an exact science on the basis of precisely calculable rational state interests.

Bismarck typifies a cleavage which is socially more significant than is the duality of the theoretical intellect and practical action drive within the occasional scholar-statesman himself. More, even, than one of cleavage, the relationship between statecraft and scholarship is one of alienation. Appearances to the contrary, that alienation is as great or greater in international politics than it is in any other area where the worlds of thought and action interact and either complement or bypass one another. Reciprocal depreciation verges on real or simulated contempt. The practitioner tends to be genuinely contemptuous of the scholar's capacity to make either a relevant or an original contribution that would be useful and usable beyond supplying rationalization and support for official policies in being or becoming. The scholar's wounded ego drives him into a basic posture of skepticism regarding the capacity and performance of the practitioners. Each side has its own particular handicap and compensations. Where the statesman must act in large ignorance of immediate responses and future developments, he can at least shape such responses and developments in part by his actions. The scholar can critically judge with fuller knowledge in retrospect, but when prescribing even but general lines of policy he has no way to validate prescription through direct (or, most of the time, indirect) impact on its adoption or implementation.

It is differences such as these in the basic predicament that engender the surface manifestations of alienation, which are then intensified in the inherently passional milieu of power and its exercise. The scholar deserves the statesman's contempt—or, worse, indifference—when he is wholly negative in the sense of being only critical; when he refuses to enter sympathetically into the statesman's perceived environment and his dilemmas and abstains from the effort of developing a complementary method and structure, however different it will be from the practitioner's in terms of both level and kind of analysis, degree of abstraction and generality, and mix of logical coherence and practical applicability. An approach that is at once sympathetic and systemic is in no way certain to catch the eye of the statesman and receive his approval as relevant. But it will insure the social utility and preserve the self-respect of the scholar-about-statecraft as one who remains in touch with significant realities in his own way: as one, that is, who contemplates the world of foreign policy through a prism essentially like that of the actors themselves, but from farther aloft. One alternative to the sympathetic-systemic approach is to trail the practitioner until he stumbles or deviates from the straight and narrow path of patent efficacity or virtue—and then announce this *urbi et orbi*, without having a sure basis for knowing whether the stumble was not a feint and the apparent deviation the politically (if not geometrically) shortest pathway to the approved goal. The other alternative is to transcend statecraft as practiced and project its works critically against radically different constructs and related standards; to view matters from on high while refusing to focus on what is actively there; to look through rather than at and, in the end, repudiate rather than criticize.

Ideally, the truth about statecraft is not in commonplace practice or in either trivial or sophisticated academic analysis. It is, once again, in a tension supplementing that between the sublime and the humdrum or trivial aspects of statecraft itself. In this case, the tension is between the pole of creative practicing statecraft and the pole of the rational scholarly reconstruction and constructive critique of statecraft's works. Occasionally, by sheer and rare accident, the tension and the resulting "truth" or "essence" of statecraft is expressed positively in the writings of the statesman-turned-scholar—a political animal that is rarer still than is its obverse when it comes to a genuinely speculative cast of mind. Machiavelli, as one who transcended in that respect both an essayist like Bolingbroke and a memorialist like Bismarck, is likely to remain the paramount example of the scholarly ex-practitioner. An intellectual process and a psychological process conspire to produce the type. The first entails the distillation in writings of past experience (filtered through historical learning), and the second, the sublimation through writing of the drive for power or just self-expression in action. To the yearning to reenter the real world by the gateway of scholarly fiction, the experience of office supplies the matter; exile from office, the leisure and the perspective; and the desire to recapture power actually or vicariously, the energy for refining practice into propositions. For the scholar lacking direct contact with great affairs, only prolonged immersion in detailed accounts of past diplomatic transactions can substitute for the experience of the statesman-turned-scholar even in part.

The ambition to act can alone give the appetite for undertaking the in itself thankless effort to convert petty transactions into treatises on the sublime and thought into a guide to more accomplished transactions. In Machiavelli's design, the excellence of his thought would recommend him for reemployment by the Prince. There are valid grounds for this pretension. The mirror which the "Machiavellian" thinker holds up for the Prince's inspection reflects the world as it is, yet reduced to a finite circumference by the very medium in which it is reflected. It is a both limited and limiting view; there is much in scope and in depth that the mirror by its very nature is unable to capture, and neither can diplomatic statecraft of the most creative kind nor scholarship-about-statecraft of the most imaginative kind. They both deal and can deal with reality only at the level where it can be sharply enough reflected in strategic thought and inflected by strategic action of a quite special kind. They, like the mirror, serve well if the image received and projected is the image of objects that are actually there and really matter and if the handle used to inflect the reflected reality in the desired direction is shaped to fit the grasp, and placed to fit the reach, of man.

III. THE BISMARCKIAN SYSTEM: THE NIXON-KISSINGER STRATEGY AND BEYOND

Anyone who wishes to seriously evaluate or perpetuate achievements of creative statecraft has to pay attention to a particular and critical fit: that between the diplomatic system (or, in the classic language of the craft, *système*) of a statesman and the international system within and with which he has to work. The first is a matter of subtle contrivances aiming at desired ends through suitable constellations; abstracted from the shaping effect of these, the second consists of the gross structures of power and conflict already in existence. The immediate profit of a diplomatic system for different parties is one thing, easily and often unfairly assessable; the master statesman's real measure is determined more accurately by his unique discernment of the right constellation and of its longer-term potentialities.

I

In classic European statecraft there were three great *systèmes*: the Kaunitzian, the Metternichian, and the Bismarckian. Their delineation ought to help evaluate recent American foreign policy at different points in time. It ought, moreover, to permit the separation of issues of diplomatic style from those of substance, sensations of the day from structures evolving over decades.

As the war-related reversal from an "old" system (of Austro-British versus Franco-Prussian alliances) into its opposite (Austro-French versus Anglo-Prussian alignments), the Kaunitzian system, while least known of the three, sets the theoretical and practical boundaries within which the Metternichian and the Bismarckian diplomatic strategies—and their approximations—cannot quite avoid evolving. The mid-eighteenth-century Austrian statesman is credited with seducing French diplomacy into the diplomatic revolution which reconciled the Habsburgs and the rival Catholic dynastic house of France, in association with Russia, as part of an unevenly shared opposition to the Protestant upstart powers of

Prussia in Europe and Britain overseas. The anticipated immediate payoff of the Kaunitzian system did not materialize for either party, as Prussia was not destroyed in Europe and Britain was not displaced in America and the Indies. Within a century, however, the fit of the *système* with the international system was demonstrated in five short years (1866–71), when the failure to revive the Franco-Austrian-Russian coalition in part or in whole resulted in the successive demotion of Austria in the Germanies and of France in Europe from their previously high estate. Bismarck himself sanctioned the posthumous vindication when he threatened the Kaiser with the revival of the "Kaunitzian coalition" should he not agree to keeping Austria away from her erstwhile allies by way of the dual Austro-German alliance. Although never effectually implemented, Kaunitz's diplomatic system is thus shown nonetheless to have been solidly grounded in the evolving structure of the international system. In brief, the structure consisted of two relatively declining and conservative powers seeking to preserve their advantageous status relative to newly ascendant states by means of compensating expansion in different directions. The directions were implicit in the dualistic structure of the dominant conflicts: one was over the intra-German (and, by extension, Continental) balance of power, the other over the colonial-maritime (and, by extension, global) balance of power. The conflicts, and resulting expansion, were compatible if both France and Austria achieved an about equal measure of success.

Transposed to the present, the Kaunitzian *système* implies a consummated diplomatic revolution—i.e., the United States abandoning or downgrading its principal alliances in favor of an integral politico-military alliance with either Soviet Russia or China aimed at the curtailment of the other and the consolidation or expansion of the victors' orbits of dominance or influence. Such a reversal could, in principle, favor Soviet Russia on historical grounds and China on geopolitical grounds: Russia was the principal enemy in the preceding cold-war era, eligible as such for a "conservative" partnership against China as the new principal disturber of the balance; conversely, China is the potentially flanking counterpoise to Soviet Russia as the centrally situated Eurasian power encroaching in both directions. To put matters this way is to suggest that the identity of neither the preferred ally nor the more provocative antagonist is self-evident; nor has an exclusive and integral alliance with one Communist great power sufficient appeal for official policy at the present juncture. One reason bears on the possible military-strategic reactions of the power selected for target of such an alliance. A related reason is that, if fully successful, the two triumphant allies would find themselves face to face across a power vacuum of a kind that had produced the cold war in the first place. There are currently no distracting powers in evidence that could replicate Russia and Britain as survivors to the elimination of Prussia as a great power in the Kaunitzian context. The victors would not, moreover, have the attenuating advantage of looking to different areas for aggrandizement as had, with qualifications, France and Austria. Could or would the United States surrender Asia to a co-triumphant Chinese ally (in exchange for Eastern Europe) any more than it could relinquish major parts of Northeast or Southeast Asia and the Middle East (in exchange for the remainders) to the Soviet partner in success? To pose the questions in such absolute terms is to answer them—without implying, however, that the absolute terms are either the only possible or the most pertinent ones.

The key quandary for a full-fledged neo-Kaunitzian diplomatic system at any later stage would be the determination of which of the two Communist powers was more congenial because internationally more conservative than the other in policies reflective of internal structures and externally usable capabilities. The query has a different meaning within a neo-Metternichian system. The most essential strand in the original model consisted of attaching Austria to a power that was more vital than the Habsburg conglomerate as a force and was equally conservative in basic policy. At first, Metternich could hope to pursue the objective while guarding intact Austria's independence as a great power (chiefly from Russian patronage) by stressing the international or balance-of-power side of conservation (against Russian expansion west- and southward). In such a context the most attractive ally was a Bonapartist France without Napoleon (under the regency of the Habsburg-born empress). Failing that too daring option, Metternich's preferred ally was a Great Britain reinvolved on the Continent in peacetime during Castlereagh's stewardship. When long-term revolutionary threats to internal social hierarchies reduced immediate threats to the equilibrium among the powers by taking precedence, and Britain again evacuated Europe diplomatically as a result, Metternich had to subordinate the value of Austria's independence in policy to her mere survival as great power in status. The principal ally in the new circumstances had to be Russia; and Metternich was compelled to set about revising secular balance-of-power calculations to fit Austria's necessity for a holy alliance for order. Side by side with the preferred-ally strand, the Metternichian *système* comprised an assiduous pursuit of diplomatic concert—or moral consensus—among all the powers. Under the cover name of legitimacy, Metternich sought concert initially as a safeguard from inimical interference for Austria's forcible interventions in areas under her hegemony (Italy and Germany). Thereafter, as Austria grew weaker and more dependent, the early preoccupation yielded to one more typical: to have Austria's waning influence enhanced by an institutionalized right of interference in matters directly concerning more independently active powers (thus in Belgium and Egypt in the 1830s).

The Metternichian diplomatic system was fundamentally in keeping with the international system. France had finally declined from continental preeminence, weakened by the profitless strains of the mismanaged Kaunitzian system and by the Napoleonic relapse into hegemonial politics. As a result, effectively usable power was more evenly diffused in Europe even while the issue of hegemony gravitated overseas. Conflicts were likewise dispersed, along the lines of conservative versus liberal ideology, and predominantly continental versus maritime power. This militated against any tendency to consolidate an east-west polarity pitting "liberal" Britain and France against the "autocratic" courts of Austria, Russia, and Prussia. A flexible situation guaranteed the continuing diplomatic utility of Austria, while no major power was tempted to pursue major goals that would put to test the military potential of the Habsburg monarchy. Inasmuch as Metternich's system was primarily intended to insure Austria's survival as the preeminent Germanic power and thus as a respectable European power, it was vindicated by Russia's support for Austria against Prussia in the aftermath of the 1848 revolution. It was, by the same standard, disastrously undermined when a successor to Metternich tried to revert to the ideal of Austrian independence from Russia in alliance with Britain and France in the diplomacy of the Crimean War. The *faux pas* caused Russia eventually to back the conversion of Prussia into Imperial Germany, which removed the foundation from the Metternichian diplomatic system by replacing Russia's patronage in Germany with Germany's preeminence in Europe.

Any literal transference of the Metternichian system would run counter to the fact that the contemporary United States is not (yet?) in the developmental stage of Austria in the age of Metternich and after. That is to say, it is not a decadent power which is, as a result, fitfully assertive and locally expansionist. The United States does not, therefore, have as vital a stake in an institutionalized concert of all great powers as the condition of diplomatic influence and occasional independence at the least cost in material exertions. But neither has power been so far diffused and conflict dispersed in more than token—or anticipatory—fashion in the contemporary international system. That system might not provide, therefore, ready alternatives to the unfolding costs of a two-power conservative alliance for the party that would be, even relatively, declining. Consequently, a U.S. policy of a too-exclusive accommodation, if not alliance, with the Soviet Union might evolve in certain circumstances in the direction of Metternich's onetime submission to Russia, which was leavened only by pretensions of personal mastery. The remotest possibility of this happening draws attention to Metternich's diplomatic style as against system. In one view, the style can be defined and distinguished by statesmanlike concern for a painstakingly evolved moral consensus among the powers as the preliminary to joint or unilateral initiatives. In another and more skeptical view, it can be reduced to a certain timidity in basic attitude toward risk and a consequent tendency to temporize and delay. It was the latter view which predominated among Metternich's contemporaries, who perceived him as either hanging back from transactions and transformations including more than routine risks or, alternatively, as making diplomatic agitation do duty for statesmanlike achievement.

An ingrained timidity would be out of keeping with American power that survived the Vietnam exertions, even if it conformed to the ensuing American mood. The power was still sufficient to make the United States resemble Bismarck's Germany more than Metternich's Austria. The shared identity is that of a preeminent power, conservative due to saturation abroad rather than decay from within: one exercising leadership in military organization and technology, even if not in all respects in capability, from a focal position in the international system—in America's case between Russia and China as either continuing rivals or reunited partners in an anti-American coalition. On the other hand, however, the international system facing Bismarck was more like that confronting Metternich than is the contemporary one. Five (or, counting Italy, six) great powers were at once divided by and clustered around several conflict axes: the Western or continental-European question (France versus Germany); the Near Eastern question (Britain and Austria versus Russia); the colonial, including Far Eastern, question (separating France from Britain); and the "revolutionary" question (dividing Russia from France). The international system had, moreover, a focus on which most or all powers could agree. The focus was still France, though henceforth only as a restlessly revisionist and residually revolutionary power —at once an irritant (to Germany and Russia on the Continent and to Britain in the colonies and overseas) and a protégé (of Russia and Britain against additional curtailment by Germany in Europe). The commonality among the powers around France facilitated Bismarck's diplomacy of counterposing the powers against one another by a combination of diplomatic intrigue and contractual instruments. Thus Britain and Austria were pitted against Russia, and both Russia and Britain and Italy against France, in function of conflicts just sufficiently intense and complementary to facilitate diplomatic constructions and avoid major military conflagrations.

The post-Vietnam international system has, by contrast, continued to display only three great powers, despite favorable prognoses for Western Europe and Japan to complete the magic five. When the Nixon-Kissinger team stressed the diffusion of military-political power in a triangular framework, this was convenient with respect to efforts at "normalizing" relations with China; the administration actually overstressed the diffusion of economic power into a pentagonal pattern as a method for revising balances of defense-costs and trade with respect to Western Europe and Japan. And even the United States, Russia, and China have not been as near-equal in power and as evenly active over comparably limited ends, with by and large equal or symmetric access to one another diplomatically, as had been the case for the powers of the earlier era save for the Franco-German schism (itself confined to European matters). The decreasingly ideological conflict between the United States and both the Soviet Union and China over the balance of power has not been either matched or displaced by newly emerging conflicts involving the three major powers and any additional great and middle powers. Only as a long-term potentiality could issues centering on economic development and both overland and maritime environment align the United States and a Russia more fully motivated by its status as an advanced industrial-maritime great power against a China that became able—or was, in the face of U.S.-Soviet solidarity, compelled—to militantly implement "revolutionary" leadership of the developing Third World. Similarly, only thus could the conflict over military-naval and related issues centered on the Indian Ocean cause America's global and China's continental preoccupations to converge against a generally ascendant Soviet Russia in an alliance going beyond *ad hoc* diplomatic alignment or concert on a particular issue.

Being deficient in complementary conflicts, the contemporary system has likewise not had much room for the kind of compensations which must complement counterpoising in the peaceful managing of conflicts. In the Bismarckian era, compensations could draw on the decaying Ottoman empire with just barely sufficient ease and ultimate concord. Today's post-imperial Third World has served the three great powers even less well as a set of either irritants or protégés focusing their diplomacy (in lieu of volatile France), or as an area of compensations (in lieu of the unspeakable Turk). This aggravated the tendency for compensations to be practically available only in previously U.S.-controlled capital assets. The further result was that the compensations of which post-Vietnam American statecraft could readily dispose tended to be individually only symbolic or spasmodic: among the symbolic ones were nuclear parity with respect to Soviet Russia and diplomatic parity in regard to China; the spasmodic ones included intermittent gestures in favor of economic credits in trade and diplomatic co-management in the Middle East with the Soviets and of disengagement in Taiwan for the potential long-term benefit of mainland China. A major reason for this has been that in the sum of their material implications, even the separately symbolic or spasmodic concessions were potentially disequilibrating and thus vulnerable to domestic criticism and opposition in the United States when their one-sided impact was not being simultaneously neutralized within a new configuration.

Limitations affecting the relations among the great powers engendered pressures and temptations to shift the technique of counterpoising and compensating ever more to contentions among lesser states: Israel versus the Arabs, Greece versus Turkey, India versus Pakistan. The resulting exercise was residually imperial relative to the small states, just as its manifestations had been *grosso modo* Bismarckian in the Nixon-Kissinger team's approach to the Communist great powers. The American diplomatic action was lowered in either quality or efficacy, however, by its deficient basis in supporting strategic imagination and capacity or will for authoritative intervention. The two deficiencies in combination augmented the limitations inherent in the desire to simultaneously further the reemergent inter-great-power cooperation for equilibrium and to competitively retain local advantages of empire.

On the most favorable view, the evolution of an equilibrium among the great powers has been occurring with glacierlike slowness as a result. It was punctuated by stoppages and setbacks that had much—but not everything—to do with the diplomatic and domestic dilemmas attending compensations and with the structural dilemma inherent in tripolarity. If continuing competition was sufficient to impede progress toward global equilibrium by virtue of authoritatively joint action with at least one Communist great power for regional order, it could even more effectively thwart unilateral mediation for regional peace among lesser-state contestants. The immediate consequence has been to deny to the initial quasi-Bismarckian Nixon-Kissinger *système* even the limited quota of consolidation at the center and ramification into the peripheries that had been achieved by Bismarck himself. Its precarious character required ever more equilibristic juggling alongside more fundamental equilibration. This fact alone seemed to strengthen the case for simplifying the "Bismarckian" diplomatic system. Short of the U.S. reverting to single-handed hegemony, greater simplicity meant retreating from Bismarck to Metternich, possibly *en route* to Kaunitz—consummating the "holy alliance" as the more or less unwitting step toward a "diplomatic revolution."

The Metternichian course meant a fuller commitment to a conservative accommodation with Soviet Russia, with a potential for superpower solidarity against any resurgence of China-backed Third-World radicalism globally or nuclear-backed assertiveness regionally. The Kaunitzian course (or Kaunitzian consequence of the Metternichian course) was implicit in opposition to an exclusive détente with the Soviet Union or in its ultimate fiasco. It would signify an "alliance" with China against a Russia that would grow or has grown too strong and expansive in traditional or conventional terms. Inflecting U.S. foreign policy away from the Bismarckian system meant thus giving up the will or ability to keep both balls—the Soviet and Chinese—in the air, or to press on both levers, at the same time or alternately, for the good of both global and regional interests. It meant that an excess of the Metternichian diplomatic style and political philosophy inhibited the director or directors of American statecraft from exploring the terrain sufficiently along the Bismarckian road while the United States could still do this from adequate basic strength.

II

In the first Nixon administration, concerned chiefly with liquidating the war in Indochina, there were grounds for comparing the dominant strategy with Bismarck's diplomatic system. This was true particularly for the relations with China and the Soviet Union. The early double triumph actually derived from the Vietnam war itself, as the new administration terminated the ostensible follies of the war in the military field and conspicuously harvested the war's hidden fruits on the diplomatic one. The harvesting occurred as the Chinese fear of an American impulse to leave Southeast Asia to the benefit of the Soviets dovetailed with the Soviet apprehension lest corrective American reactions to that impulse unduly reinforce the Chinese. The leverage that was implicit in the mining of Haiphong and the reintensified bombing in North Vietnam helped midwife both the American military withdrawal from Indochina and the American diplomatic progress to a new type of relations with the Communist great powers. The last-ditch military measures were both a warning and an inducement to those powers, and they were acceptable to them because the United States escalated force while local "Vietnamization" and the enunciation of the more far-reaching "Nixon Doctrine" signaled its engagement in a fundamental course of withdrawal from furthermost American advance in the area. The Nixonian mix thus combined tactical self-assertion with strategic retreat. This was the exact opposite of the Johnson formula at its apogee. Both presidents desired the same thing in regard to Soviet Russia and Communist China, but Johnson's searing disappointments only prepared the soil from which was to sprout the climactic accomplishment of the Nixon-Kissinger team.

Insofar as it consisted of playing off the two Communist great powers against one another, triangular diplomacy comprised the great-power dimension of the Bismarckian diplomatic system. That statecraft has, however, two major components. Both of them involve finding and then occupying a place somewhere between strenuous hegemony and paralyzing deadlock. One strand of the system has to do with constellations among the great powers. It involves reciprocally counterpoising these powers in such a way as to reduce the surviving margin of usable power and effectively inimical purpose to a manageable dimension at any one time. The other strand concerns crises and conflicts in the international system. It involves imposing oneself as the mediating honest broker to powers more directly concerned. If the two strategies are successful, they add up to a kind of preeminence on the cheap. A secure leadership in equilibrium diplomacy rests, then, mainly on one's superiority in available options; and it absolutely requires no more than parity in the supporting military stalemate.

The great-power strand has an immediate specific objective which concerns war. Its more general and longer-term purpose is concerned with consolidaing one's position in a stabilized environment. In Bismarck's case, this meant first of all isolating Prussia's adversaries in the two wars of German unification. Subsequently, it meant preventing the rivals of imperial Germany from finding common ground for a grand coalition against the consequences of German unification for the European balance of power. For the Nixon administration, the power to be at least partially isolated in war by great-power diplomacy from all-out outside support was North Vietnam. The long-term task was to forestall a voluntary or imposed re-coalescence of China with Soviet Russia. Both objects could be pursued simultaneously by moving the United States into the posture of a partial-potential ally for China in particular and by improving relations with both Communist powers in general. The basic condition of the second, conflict-moderation strand is that the mediatory power be recognized as either "omnipotent" or "objective." That is to say, it must be either capable of imposing not only its services but also its solution, or else must be wholly disinterested in the critical area of contention. The specific requirement, especially in the second case, is that the contentious parties are looking for a way out that would save face and reduce costs when compared with continuing and intensifying the conflict.

The difference between Bismarck and the Nixon-Kissinger team in the great-power arena involves the magnitude of immediate achievement. Out of unformed elements, Bismarck evolved in succession great-power constellations enabling Prussia to win two wars and rise to settled continental preeminence with the support or toleration of both of the serious long-term rivals, Russia and Britain. By contrast, Nixon and Kissinger merely surfaced a latent configuration that had been widely perceived and favored before. They did so with powerful aid from the Vietnam war itself, which served as a crystallizer of trends and remover of oppositions, internal American as well as Chinese. In a yet undefinable complementary relationship, Nixon and Kissinger converted a long-drawn-out organic evolution within the Communist powers and the international system into the beginnings of a revolution both diplomatic and systemic. They did not create, as did Bismarck, both its conditions and its contours out of near-nothing by reaching beyond dominant modes of thinking to an earlier tradition. The fact that the adjustments occurred as part of a retreat from global American predominance would magnify the achievement only if that retreat had not been, as it was, the essential precondition of an effective shift in the diplomatic gears that had previously been absent.

In the area of conflict moderation, Bismarck's task was by contrast the easier one of the two. Not without costs for himself and Germany, he acted as the self-styled honest broker among settled great powers, from a position of freshly acquired central strength and in an attitude of disinterest for the area of contest (what was then called the Near East, which was unworthy—in Bismarck's words—of the bones of a single Pomeranian grenadier). The real or pretended reduction of the United States from empire to equilibrium lowered American self-perception as omnipotent, and it helped enhance the inclination to be objective in regard to peripheral conflicts of lesser powers—and even to be perceived as such from the outside. But the partial retreat did not bestow upon American statecraft either the feeling or the presumption of disinterest in areas of continuing, if muted, competition with one or both of the Communist great powers. Only such disinterest might, however, have enabled the United States to enjoy effortlessly the complete confidence of all local parties (and toleration by interested outside parties) as the impartial mediator and reliable guarantor, even while reducing its incentives to undertake the effort. What mattered decisively, henceforth, was the degree to which the local parties were, and continued to be, eager to be helped out of an oppressive conflict or to escape or avoid a burdensome alignment. Much as the condition was initially present in the Middle East on the part of Egypt and Israel following the October war in 1973, its very precarious character was liable to make any mediatory successes likewise precarious and reversible —and difficult to extend beyond the stage of an immediate political and military easement in any but uniquely and lastingly propitious circumstances. A more reliable strategy for more enduring success would depend, consequently, on combining both of the strands—mediatory and constellating—in one coherent strategy for regional peace and global stability.

Such a combination has not been forthcoming from an American statecraft undergoing a sea change at a point roughly coinciding with the decay of the second Nixon administration and Kissinger's ascent to primacy in the making of foreign policy. The change may have been intended from the beginning—an intention that would reduce the "opening" to China to the level of Nixon's flirt with Rumania as the tactical device for softening up Soviet Russia for inter-superpower accommodation. Or the change in policy may have reflected a change in effective command and control over that policy. By shifting from effective triangular diplomacy to two-power détente, Kissinger seemed to jettison the Bismarckian strategy on the great-power level while seeking to perpetuate the mediatory role in lesser-power conflict as part of the newly intensified needs and opportunities in the Middle East. It cannot be decided from the outside how much Kissinger, in so doing, followed his philosophic biases and how much he was bowing before the limitations that the lopsided and truncated structure of power and conflicts in the *international* system implied for the Bismarckian *diplomatic* system. In any event, he renounced a creative effort to narrow the gap between the two kinds of systems. That is to say, by singling out the Soviet Union as the altogether primary object of concern, he downgraded the effort to promote either multilateralization of power or diversification of conflicts (to be distinguished from their diminution) on either the great- or the middle- and small-power levels. To appreciate the degree of inflection that occurred and the kind of diplomatic system which was actually pursued, it will be useful first to illustrate a manipulative or Bismarckian type of diplomatic strategy for relations with both great and small powers that was *not* in evidence and then to delineate the conservative détente and peacemaking strategies which Kissinger actually followed as secretary of state.

Put most succinctly and schematically, a Bismarckian strategy for a United States retreating from empire to equilibrium implied a continuing and active effort to (1) keep China in the triangular game and (2) move Western Europe and Japan into a more active role in the international politics of the balance of power. The object of a developing China connection would be to both contain and control the tempo of Soviet ascent in general and to promote *ad hoc* concert with the Soviet Union on specific issues, including regional peace settlements. A partial activation of Western Europe and Japan, while being itself a near-automatic response to the complete activation of China, might likewise facilitate instances of U.S.-Soviet entente. Specifically, one or both of the principal U.S. allies would constitute an additional counterpoise to the Soviet Union when they had become more active and self-reliant; but, crucial from the Chinese perspective, they could also supplement whatever diminution in direct American constraint on the Soviet Union might result from a specific U.S.-Soviet entente on a particular issue or a general détente. The result would be an at least marginally multilateralized triangular system. It would be consolidated when a diplomatically fully integrated and strategically reassured China had every incentive not to dilute her full great-power status in a re-formed Sino-Soviet alliance and no incentive to pursue such status by intensifying "revolutionary" diplomacy.

As a power standing at the center of the equilibrium system, the United States would occupy and could gradually consolidate a leadership role. A stabilized equilibrium system must be distinguished from surface stability due to mere momentary absence of active conflict. To pursue stability in depth would require relating the great-power level to (1) peacemaking in the immediately disturbed areas such as Southeast Asia and the Middle East and (2) to crystallizing regional orders in fragmented areas such as South Asia. The general objective would be to complement in the lesser-power arenas the basic strategy (of counterpoising) and structure (of a hierarchically stratified balance-of-power system) that was already incipiently in existence among the greater powers themselves. A complex two-tier system would tend to be structurally stable. It would also be operationally stable if the United States, as the equilibrium leader, could competitively evolve complementary ties or *ad hoc* concerts with both of the Communist great powers in different areas—e.g., with China in Southeast or South Asia and with the Soviet Union in the Middle East.

The most effective method for involving China actively in global great-power diplomacy was by way of peacemaking for the region closest to her in immediate interest. Such involvement might, moreover, have facilitated the regional political settlement itself. One premise is that involving both of the Communist great powers in regional settlements and linking the strategy for Southeast Asia with peacemaking in the Middle East (and vice versa) would have usefully enlarged the overall field of forces, expanded the range of available leverages, and created additional room for demonstrations of capability and intent as well as for specific *quid-pro-quo* barters between the regions. The other basic premise bears on the regional actors. It holds that a relatively peaceful settlement in Southeast Asia depended on managing the process of North Vietnam's ascent to some form of *political* hegemony in Indochina, once American intervention had failed to insure a stable south-north military equilibrium in Vietnam; and that peacemaking in the Middle East required the "threat" of U.S. backing for some form of Israeli *military* hegemony in the region in order to achieve an equilibrium solution politically.

Proceeding from the two basic premises, it is possible to speculate about appropriate strategies. One possibility worth exploring in the wake of the Vietnam cease-fire was (and continued to be for a time with diminishing chance of success) to seek the active support of one of the Communist great powers, acting in competition with the other, for an American policy to circumscribe an overall Hanoi preponderance in either Vietnam or Indochina as a whole, while conceding it. The hegemony—implemented through some form of coalition government in the South—would reflect the military conclusions in the field. Its confinement short of total dominance (and destruction of all non-Communist political forces in the South) would reflect the new kind of Washington-Hanoi relations that had been wrought by the war and the agreements terminating mutual belligerence. The new conditions comprised, next to its need for the pledged American assistance for reconstruction, Hanoi's even more permanent need for political aid toward independence from both of the Communist great powers. As a result of the war it became more readily possible for the United States, and quite possibly more necessary for Hanoi, to do what the war's critics in the United States mistakenly deemed feasible before and without America's involvement in the war. Moreover, it remained within the power of the United States to make Hanoi's self-limitation reflect the residual American capacity to either oppose or punish forcefully a too-crude and precipitate drive to foreshorten the unfolding of historical necessity in Indochina. Such capacity would be strengthened if Hanoi acted to overthrow previously agreed-upon and implemented political structures and arrangements. For the same domestic political reasons, the American capacity to act forcefully has become easier to revive and demonstrate in the Middle East than in Southeast Asia. Hence the desirability to continue incessantly the search for a political settlement in Southeast Asia following the cease-fire and to interrelate it with the quest for peace in the area of the Arab-Israeli conflict.

In different circumstances, either conflict or concert with the Soviet Union was the more promising avenue to the goal of a limited and safeguarded Hanoi supremacy. Intensified conflict with Moscow was liable to shift China toward the side of the American effort as the only way to undercut Soviet influence in Hanoi, which was contingent on Hanoi's continuing need for massive supplies of arms in an unresolved situation. Conversely, an *ad hoc* Soviet-American concert on Indochina would become possible whenever the Soviets preferred positive cooperation with the United States to serious American-Soviet confrontation or far-reaching American-Chinese understanding. American-Soviet concert on Indochina could be an extension, or even the stipulated *quid pro quo*, of a like concert for a political settlement in the Middle East. Or, again, concert between the United States and China over Southeast Asia could be expected to encourage the Soviet Union to contain its ramifications by moving closer to the United States on the Middle East. Alternatively, concert with China in the Soviets' Asian rear would insure, and might procure active support for, an American confrontation with the Soviet Union in the Middle East. Such a confrontation is the predictable concomitant of a peace strategy for the Middle East that is keyed to a regional Arab-Israeli equilibrium guaranteed by the United States alone, or that is forced by hostile Arab responses into underwriting a circumscribed Israeli military hegemony; and it may also be the necessary preliminary to a concert.

Concert with the Soviets in the Middle East would tend toward an equilibrium solution for the Middle East imposed and supervised by both superpowers. Concert with either of the Communist great powers in Southeast Asia implied limitation on local hegemony for Hanoi. As long as fighting continued in Indochina (and in a much weakened and different mode thereafter), the fact or prospect of either an American-Soviet or an American-Chinese concert threatened to reduce Hanoi to undesired dependence on the Communist great power that was excluded from the two-power concert. In order to avoid this, Hanoi might well have been—or might eventually again become—receptive to accommodation with the United States on the basis of less far-reaching and immediate gains that might be achieved hypothetically in violent opposition to the United States and in integral servitude to the Communist sponsor. Roughly the same reaction could be anticipated from the more moderate and sophisticated Arab adversaries of Israel. It would tend to separate them from the all-out radicals, who would be weakened in any event if America's concert partner in Asia were to be China.

A possible local cost of American-Soviet conflict would be compensation for China in Southeast Asia (more immediately in Cambodia than with respect to Taiwan?). An American-Soviet concert might well either solidify Soviet presence in one part of the Middle East (insofar as condominium tends to rest on separate spheres of influence for each of the co-guarantors) or else diffuse a diluted Soviet influence more widely (to encompass Israel). The United States would gain too, however, as would the local parties, from inflecting the political track in peacemaking along with the military one toward local appeasement.

By contrast, the costs of avoiding both conflict and concert with either of the Communist great powers have been several. The United States shrank from playing a stronger hand in either the Middle East or Southeast Asia also for fear of disrupting the delicate, if sterile, policy of limited competition and cooperation. Both of the Communist powers had reason to avoid antagonizing Hanoi, which remained crucial for them as the effective reserve asset against one another and as the potential pressure point on a United States that only might defect too far to the other great power at some future date. The U.S. policy of neither-conflict-nor-concert encouraged the Soviet Union to straddle the differences between moderates and radicals in the Middle East as a likewise necessary precaution in an indeterminate and protracted situation. Specifically, neither of the Communist great powers had a motive for restricting Hanoi's leeway for reintensified military activities in the short run any more than it had one for aiding the United States directly or indirectly in confining the leeway of the Arabs for eroding the Israeli security position by politico-economic and paramilitary means in the longer run.

It was not necessarily an accident that Hanoi unleashed—or was unleashed for—its military push in early 1975, just as a publicly resentful Moscow was putting an end to its prior exclusion from the Middle Eastern peacemaking by Kissinger's step-by-step approach and China's premier spokesman was reaffirming world revolutionary themes to avoid falling behind. As military conditions in Cambodia and South Vietnam deteriorated dramatically, it was increasingly difficult to admit that the overt American exertions prior to the Paris accords, and the more or less covert commitments on the military plane attendant on those accords, ought not to have been complemented on the political stage by continuing equivalent exertions and, if the painful and unglorious necessity arose, overt and manifest concessions for corresponding adjustments. In the absence of such efforts in comparatively still-favorable military contexts, it became ever more difficult to resist arguments against continuing the expenditure of resource and credit associated with the military dimension in isolation—one day in Indochina, another day in the Middle East.

A broadly identical, Bismarckian type of diplomatic strategy could be applied more widely to the development of regional orders based on local balance-of-power systems. Applying that kind of strategy for the politically more active and exposed Third-World regions does not postulate as immediately feasible or desirable either regional associations of local states, on the basis of political equality and cooperation for economic and political ends, or the dissociation of great powers from regional politics and conflicts. It postulates, that is, neither depoliticization nor neutralization of such regions. Instead, manipulative statecraft for regional equilibrium systems presupposes the existence of what actually is, or is likely to become, the case over a short-to-medium term. One supposition is that conflicts will occur in some regions or in different regions alternately and will revolve around both material and status issues (both territory and other specific assets and degrees of local ascendancy and subordination); and even relatively quiescent areas where such issues had been previously settled or have not yet arisen will be involved in the ferment by the ripple effect of conflicts in adjacent areas to a degree that may initiate sustained inter-regional equilibrium politics.

Local conflicts and their ramifications will occasion, and may necessitate, involvement in balancing or counterpoising activities by both regional and extra-regional states of different magnitudes. In the process, some of the great powers will express support for ascendant or assertive regional middle powers as a matter of fundamental sympathy with the latter's role in crystallizing regional balance-of-power orders and assuming greater responsibility for regional order—or else as a matter of expediency dictated by the interested great power's own global strategy relative to its peers. At other points, the great powers will oppose too-assertive middle powers either in cooperation with other intra- or extra-regional middle powers or by supporting the small regional states in their effort to eschew the conversion of a middle power's regional pre-eminence (or hegemony) into unrestrained local dominance. "Hegemony" may be constituent of a regional balance-of-power system in its beginnings and may be compatible with intra-regional equilibrium when such a system is linked to complementary ones in adjacent regions or among the great powers globally. "Dominance" is neither, when it had eliminated all possibility of local resistance and independence of the smaller states and of all, including indirect, reinforcement of them.

A certain flexibility or elasticity will be introduced into regional situations insofar as a rebound syndrome complements the ripple effect and facilitates the redressal of too-lopsided local power structures by virtue of alignments or strategies involving the great powers. The ripple effect means that locally weakened states may hope to get sufficient reinforcement from the adjoining region by the play of the adjoining balance-of-power system to be able to resist and confine one-power local supremacy, even if not to wholly reverse the local power distribution. Thus Pakistan was definitively subdued in the 1971 war with India and debarred from the pursuit of anything like parity with India in the South Asian subcontinent. But, until even these conflicts have been finally composed, Pakistan remains eligible for reinforcement by an Islamic alliance with Iran in function of Iran's differences with Arab powers in the Persian Gulf area, be it with Iraq involved with the Soviet Union or Saudi Arabia leaning to the United States. Or, alternatively, Pakistan might be indirectly strengthened if an unfolding of the balance-of-power system in Southeast Asia, with or without a Chinese role, were to increase pressures on India from the east sufficiently to make India seek an accommodation with Pakistan rather than a further diminution and neutralization of Pakistan in alliance with Afghanistan or entente with Iran.

The involvement of China in Southeast Asia and of the Soviet Union in the Persian Gulf gives sufficient incentive to the other Communist power, and to the United States, to keep involved, too. All great powers can, in the postulated situation, depend on *ad hoc* "allies," both as a result of the interaction among middle and small states intra- and inter-regionally and as the middle powers rebound from an earlier great-power associate—not least one that had promoted their initial ascent to middle-power status. The rebound syndrome worked initially against the United States as the promoter of decolonization for potential middle powers, such as Indonesia under Sukarno and Egypt under Nasser; more recently, it has worked against the Soviet Union: conspicuously with Mao's China and with Sadat's Egypt, while encompassing Indonesia and some of the radical African states such as Ghana through the mechanism of internal upheavals. A North Vietnam, once it has become dominant in Indochina with the support of the Communist great powers, is liable to follow the same path if prevailing relations with the United States permit it; and only extreme Soviet caution in reacting with self-restraint to dismissal—or dismissals —from Egypt has so far precluded a similar reaction to Soviet presence in India. The Soviet position in India would become more precarious if intensified Chinese pressure from the north or the ripple effect from west or east were to force India into still-greater dependence on the Soviets. By the same token, Iran may increasingly diversify great-power ties in the direction of the Soviets as it grows in regional ascendancy with United States support and, possibly, runs up against reactions from a still more U.S.-oriented Saudi Arabia. Similarly, Turkey might diversify toward the Middle Eastern powers and the Soviet Union itself in response to U.S. constraints on its regional ambitions in Cyprus.

In such circumstances, a Bismarckian statecraft would look to equilibrium leadership for the United States based on evenhandedness between the Communist great powers and hierarchization within the regional balance-of-power systems. China can put strains on a one-sided U.S.-Soviet détente (perceived as collusion) by tightening Soviet-Indian ties due to previously intensified conventional military pressure on India from the north and revolutionary pressure on India from Southeast Asia or even via the Mideast and Persian Gulf areas. A China that has been involved constructively in political settlement in one of the critical wing regions, and placed on a par with the Soviet Union system-wide, is least likely to do so. It is thus through policy with China that the United States can be most helpful to India, albeit indirectly. Being so helpful is consistent with containing India's domineering ambitions in the subcontinent in support of a viable Pakistan, as a basis for an India-centered regional equilibrium within a larger geopolitical compass including the other local states and an India-focused inter-regional equilibrium including the two wing regions. Likewise, excessively hostile reactions to U.S.-administered constraints on Indian preeminence would warrant U.S. strategies calculated to increase pressure on India from either of the possible directions that would provisionally deepen India's involvement with the Soviet Union and would thus accelerate the pressures for rebound and consequent restraint.

As it has been developing, the new post–cold-war situation has eliminated the basic reasons for doctrinal opposition to lesser-power regional expansionism by the United States and to alignment with a great power, notably with the United States, by the middle powers. Thus, to stay with India, Nehru rejected alliance with the United States because it would reflect the global East-West conflict alien to India; would be both permanent and unequal; and would reduce India to an intolerable equality in status with, say, Ceylon, within an alliance structure polarized between the American alliance-leader and his dependent clientele. The situation changes when the management of dependent allies or regional economic communities has given way to manipulation of regional balance-of-power contests. In the politics of a regionally deconcentrated global equilibrium, alignments between great and middle powers are, or would be, made almost by definition over evolving regional and inter-regional issues. They are thus indigenous in impetus, temporary in duration, and intrinsically stratified in structure. They entail a privileged higher status for the middle-power allies relative to local smaller states regardless of whether the medium-sized powers are partners in alignments involving great powers, or their objects. As a result, the new situation eliminates the systemic sources of resentment and resistance to great-power involvement in Third-World politics. The change opens up unprecedented opportunities for manipulative statecraft of the Bismarckian type, which match the requirement for involvement by great powers on the grounds of either world order or specific national interests unavoidably affected by world-wide developments. Both opportunities and necessities increase as regional balance-of-power systems extend or ramify horizontally on the inter-regional plane or vertically between regional and global planes—thus, for instance, when the Pakistan-India interplay extends to both wing regions and all three great powers; that between Greece and Turkey, to the Arab powers (via Turkey), and to the Soviet Union (via Makarios's tactics for the Cypriote Greeks). The potential of manipulative diplomacy is inhibited, however, when domestic sympathies assert themselves as survivals from past concerns or as extensions of ethnic politics. This happens, for instance, when American sympathy for India prevails over Pakistan's self-defense needs, or political support for Greece militates against Turkey, in disregard of both the internal requirements of the diplomatic strategy and of inherent relative merit—thus India's attitude toward Kashmir has been quite similar to Turkey's on Cyprus, while eliciting different domestic and congressional responses in the United States.

Kissinger's statecraft suffered from domestic rigidities in the internationally desultory handling of the Cyprus conflict beginning with the summer of 1974. It seemed to implement support for a minimum regional balance-of-power situation when the Ford administration rescinded the embargo on arms supplies to Pakistan in early 1975. The resupply could be seen as an extension of the policy underlying the U.S. naval deployment during the 1971 war, rationalized at the time as a safeguard against the possibility of India's ambitions going beyond military defeat for Pakistan to its political dismemberment (while adjoining U.S. naval to China's verbal diplomacy on Pakistan's side as a prelude to U.S.-Chinese normalization). However, Kissinger rejected as "unacceptable" the description by Indian officials of the more recent U.S. step as being based on the "concept of . . . balance of power."[1]

If this casts doubt on the above interpretation, it has been no easier to determine what was more generally the basic strategy of the Nixon-Kissinger team, and later Kissinger's own, for giving the lesser states in the third world a "stake" in the international system and for promoting "structures of peace" there. Was the United States in favor of regional associations, hierarchically stratified

---

[1] Indian ambassador to the United States, echoing the official governmental line as reported in the *New York Times*, February 27, 1975, p. 2.

balance-of-power systems, or something different from both? The uncertainty may have been due to insufficiency of occasions, which was in turn due to the slow crystallization of local inter-state conflicts and the slow emergence of politically active middle powers (also in Africa and Latin America) resulting from the influence of either the still-salient Indochina and Arab-Israeli conflicts, the only gradual unscrambling of domestic conflicts, or the "new" and changing economic issues as provisionally dominant. Only continued U.S. interest in naval deployments—notably in the Indian Ocean—has indicated continuing interest in positions that would in principle permit pursuing either of the two basic, associational and equilibrium strategies toward lesser Third-World powers in an even interaction with the more proximate Communist great powers. A withdrawal into offshore naval strategy, hinged on small-island bases on the pattern of Diego Garcia, might, however, also mean in practice that the desirable relaxing of automatic interference with local or regional developments—characteristic of the era of the cold war and the U.N. cease-fire orders—would go too far. That is to say, it would go to the undesirable extreme of forgoing the possibility (and signaling the lack of intention?) of containing evolving local power distributions directly or indirectly within the bounds defined by the vital and manageable distinction between mere preeminence and outright domination of regional middle powers. This would mean that an intensified naval engagement in nuclear-strategic deterrence and in the defense of economic-commercial access would go hand in hand with a navally contrived dissociation from regional political developments. A continued need for in-shore facilities would militate against such total dissociation; on the other hand, an elastic balance-of-power politics for the Third World will be likewise dependent on a corresponding flexibility in the realm of naval facilities based in middling and small states.

The U.S. naval presence in the Indian Ocean could also be seen as a symbolic reassurance to China of protection against Soviet naval encirclement anchored in Somalia and India. This was, however, an at best tenuous exception to the general posture of the late-Kissingerian statecraft. Whether or not that statecraft was attuned to regional hierarchization, it did not practice anything like even-handedness in the attention given to the two Communist great powers on the global level in the aftermath of the initial diplomatic normalization with China and the military disengagement in Indochina. As secretary of state, Kissinger failed to visibly proceed to creatively develop and consolidate the triangular pattern—e.g., by way of involving both of the Communist great powers in interlocking Middle Eastern and Southeast Asian settlements—and to begin extending the triangular in the direction of the "pentagonal" (i.e., five-sided) pattern of diplomacy with military overtones, as distinct from its previously officially enunciated economic dimension. Instead, Kissinger appeared to settle for the conservative strategy of stabilizing relations with the Soviet Union on the basis of two-power détente.

IV. THE METTERNICHIAN SYSTEM: KISSINGER'S CONSERVATIVE DESIGN

In view of the great stress on its basis in philosophical doctrine and its bias toward stabilization conceived as repose, the conservative strategy reminiscent of Metternich's invites the alternative description of "design." This is also due to its being related to the ultimate goal or final consummation, and to basic trends, more tenaciously than to any particular strategic measures for getting "from here to there." To say so much is not the same, however, as to argue that the conservative design has no strategic dimension at all.

I

In a favorable interpretation, Kissinger's conservative strategy —or design—has had one central object: to reduce the scope of any devolution from the previously held American (imperial) positions to the benefit of either major allies, major adversaries, or of Third-World middle powers, while reducing the costs of upholding essential American interests. This would, ideally, be achieved by means of a diplomatic system that (1) fitted the lopsided tripolar —and, ultimately, still bipolar—structure of the international system as well as the domestic mood in the United States in favor of effective economy and an at least apparent retrenchment; and (2) would indefinitely postpone any more substantial restructuring of U.S. positions until stabilized relations between the two superpowers have minimized the twin dangers of transitional instability and temporary power vacuums.

To implement the central objective, the conservative design has had three basic components. The first of these—U.S.-Soviet détente—was to initiate newly privileged relations with the other superpower, while being designed for but a limited reach: appeasement in attitudes; progressive enmeshment of the two superpowers in a network of specific agreements, including functional and economic ones, that would engender stakes in the new stability for the Soviet Union; and a lowering of the level of military-strategic deterrence through strategic arms-limitation agreements (SALT). More far-reaching or basic forms of cooperation, in the maintenance of regional order and peace, for example, were meanwhile effectively circumscribed by the explicit bias in the Kissinger strategy against changes in the *status quo* that would even remotely raise the prospect of dominance by the Soviets in any one regional theater. Pushed to the extreme, such opposition practically nullified any general declaratory policy in support of joint conflict management, such as the Moscow Declaration of 1972. It also seriously qualified the practical significance of Kissinger's general philosophic posture of acceptance with respect to changes in the distribution of power. The second component was continued and undiminished primacy—describable as "control" or "hegemony" —of the United States in relations with its principal allies in Western Europe and Japan. The cohesion of the American alliance system was seen as the necessary prerequisite to a viable détente system and any future negotiations implementing détente (such as negotiations about European security and mutual force reductions). The third, and less important, component was the desire to see that no vacuum actually created in the Third World by U.S. disengagement—specifically in Southeast Asia—be filled by either a Communist great power, a regional middle power, or any other force other than one sanctioned or tolerated by the United States.

So interpreted, the basic conservative design was the paradoxical one of retaining the "essential" empire at a low cost with the aid of the principal suspect aspirant to imperial succession. The reduction of costs would operate in all areas: lower defense cost as a result of explicit arms-control agreements with the Soviet Union and tacit agreements on reductions in competitive foreign aid in the Third World; greater direct or indirect allied contribution against U.S. costs in performing its security role, in a context upstaging the balances of trade and payments as mechanisms coequal and conjoined with the balances of power and deterrence; and savings in the Third World by reductions in both expenditures for aid and exertions for intervention. All this would be achieved while avoiding the costs of a major systemic restructuring and devolution of influence to other powers. Soviet cooperation with this strategy would be secured by a combination of material and ideal inducements: the first in the area of technology transfers and commercial credits; the second in the form of concessions of status and legitimacy. Both of these would ideally, if now from the Soviet viewpoint, narrow the gap between the United States and the Soviet Union while widening that between the Soviet Union and China. Just as the United States would defer more fundamental political disengagement and devolution, so the Soviet Union would defer a fundamental challenge for displacing the United States as the preeminent political (as distinct from military) power. Ideally, the deferrals would be coincident in time and complementary in effect; and the challenge might never occur, either because détente transformed Soviet dispositions positively or because the structures of power were transformed so as to negate any far-reaching Soviet ambitions. Thus resurgence by aggressive China could propel détente into the completed "diplomatic revolution" of a defensive U.S.-Soviet alliance; or strengthened and matured third powers, including China, could relieve the United States in time of the monopoly in deterrence vis-à-vis the Soviet Union in favor of multi-power equilibrium dynamics. Either a peacefully stable world or a diplomatically agile (Bismarckian or Kaunitzian) world would be thus found at the end of the rainbow. This would complete the circle begun when the Bismarckian curtain-raiser for conflict termination in the first Nixon administration introduced an essentially Metternichian drama of international conservation from a position of American domestic-political weakness and conventional-military paralysis.

II

In the actual world, the implementation of the low-cost conservative design assumed progressively ever less impressive outward forms, as the initial first steps toward a diplomatic revolution world-wide tended to subside into step-by-step diplomacy in one particular region, and as the era of creativity apparently gave way to mundane caretaking. As unimpressive as such manifestations have been, and as rapidly as the superficial criticisms attending them have grown, the really critical issues were hidden in the structural and strategic foundations of the conservative design and in their relations to the presiding philosophy.

Thus, on the level of the great powers, Kissinger's handling of détente in general and of the conflicts in the Middle East and Southeast Asia in particular failed to either test or advance the constellation which emerged from the Vietnam war. Post-Vietnam American foreign policy was premised instead on the compatibility of a developing American-Soviet détente with an essentially static American-Chinese normalization and an unruffled normalcy in America's relations with Western Europe and Japan. In actuality, however, the Soviets have been enervated by Kissinger's unilateral diplomacy in the Middle East and by congressional constraints on the economic aspects of détente. The Chinese reacted unfavorably to Kissinger's failure to implement the new diplomacy conclusively in Asia (on the Taiwanese issue as well as the Indochinese one) even while he failed to demonstrate a sustained firmness in the Middle East. Such firmness, however much the Chinese might excoriate it in public (e.g., if and when brought to bear on the oil issue), would carry with it a private reassurance for China in Asia in case of renewed need (on the Sino-Soviet border issue and the nuclear issue). Conversely, the Europeans were not sufficiently reassured by the new flexibilities to eschew a show of alarm at every surface resurgence of American determination. As initiative was ebbing away from America in Asia, the Chinese have been slowly fading again as a practically significant weight in the balance. They were apparently uncertain whether a locally sterile normalization with an America subsiding on both conventional and nuclear-strategic planes into the posture of a henceforth real "paper tiger" ought not to yield priority to one with the both reascendant and seemingly conciliatory Soviets. As if by compensation for the waning elsewhere, finally, the American initiative waxed in the Atlantic region without being of a kind to jolt the Europeans into one more try at becoming a significant weight themselves.

The situation of neither war nor peace that was gradually reestablished in the Middle East after the 1973 round has been at least in part the offshoot of Kissinger's posture of neither conflict nor concert with the Communist powers in general and with the Soviet Union in particular. Nor could that posture fail to affect the reescalating prevalence of war over peace in Southeast Asia. With the exception of the SALT agreements, Kissinger's diplomacy with the Communist powers seemed to shift increasingly from the quest for major realizations to the indulgence of routine. Sales of wheat and visits to capitals were among the chosen instruments for a superficially stabilizing appeasement. The diplomacy was no more original than it promised to be effective. The "wheat" component resuscitated the policy of food without force, which has been the instinctive recourse of a practically disarmed American statecraft whenever anxious for reprieve from harsher conflict; and the "visits" carried on the diplomacy of supposedly exceptional personal rapports as a force for peace. The insufficiency of the food leverage, reminiscent of Herbert Hoover's early efforts to stem "revolution" after the First World War, was reconfirmed when it was dusted off briefly for the purposes of the lesser-power oil front; the ultimate futility of the itinerant personality factor was demonstrated by Nixon in his second term and, before that, by Eisenhower when the Dulles component had been amputated in the last phase of his administration. Kissinger's own experience conformed increasingly to the norm with the fading of the strategic leverages available for use in Nixon's first term.

In the stress on routine diplomacy for appeasement, less dramatic and more circuitous approaches to more basic stability were being neglected. Such policies would have included prompting the principal Western European allies along the path of action that might infuse real political and military (as well as economic) substance into forms of their collective identity. There was no other way for them to elude what were henceforth not two but three actual or potential "hegemonies": military Soviet, political American, *and* "Arab" economic. Instead, Kissinger inclined to alternately hectoring the allies over their best efforts and sheltering them from worst emergencies. In the tripartite relationship among the so-called limited adversaries, long-term stabilization meant different things for the two Communist powers. It meant, first of all, not allowing the China option to atrophy at the highest level, right after Vietnam, into functions more social than political, as if intermittent formal courtesies could substitute for a continuous probing for complementary capabilities and policies across the range of issues, from nuclear-strategic to geopolitical, from Eastern Europe to the Indian Ocean and the China Sea. Only the more substantive efforts held out the prospect of impressing the Soviets while holding the Chinese over time to a steadier course between alternately charging inveterate American-Soviet collusion (when reaffirming Third-World leadership in revolutionary diplomacy) and forecasting inevitable American-Soviet conflict (when resuming equidistance from both the superpowers in conventional diplomacy and disengaging from the American protector in the implicitly downgraded Sino-Soviet hostility). Furthermore, stabilization in depth meant cultivating persistently the briefly famed strategy of "linkages" between asymmetrical Soviet and American needs and assets in the various functional sectors as well as interests and goals in the various geopolitical regions. This had to be done with a visibility of means and results just sufficient to prevent the apparent disuse of the strategy in executive diplomacy from prompting its overuse in senatorial pseudo-diplomacy. It was possible to rank the damage to surface relations with the Soviet Union ensuing from senatorial initiatives no higher than the comparable gains from executive efforts. The more important damage flowed from compounding with internal derangements in constitutional responsibilities any ongoing deterioration in America's position in the overall balance of power; beyond a certain point, however, it was self-serving for the executive to impugn the domestic disorder as the uncaused cause of external setbacks and debilitation.

Intermittent spells of conflict will test the scope of effective rapprochement in the first, active phase. They are apt to advance such rapprochement in the second, reactive phase as both sides prefer reconvergence to drifting ever farther apart. Along with selectively prolonging conflict, an effective probing and promotion of desired trends will also require the statesman to employ suitable opportunities for strikingly short-cutting the avenues to *ad hoc* concert. In fact, to modulate conflict and concert at a distance from the brink has become *the* indispensable art of post–cold-war diplomacy. The profoundest implications are domestic. It will be the all-important morale of the less tightly controlled or intrinsically less disciplined of two societies which will suffer more from an indeterminate détente posture which studiously avoids applying pressure for positive change as well as paying the price of consolidation.

In connection with the October War of 1973 in the Middle East, for instance, a more convincing American push for concert in peacemaking with the Soviet Union had some potential for consolidating the American-Soviet détente and moving it toward entente on a particular issue. Any test of Soviet détente-mindedness administered in good faith had to comprise placing before the Soviet leadership (during Kissinger's lightning visit to Moscow antecedent to both cease-fire and confusion?) the outline of a political settlement. The terms of the settlement had to be such, moreover, that the Soviets could barter within them a reduction of peacetime influence for its stabilization with American endorsement and support as one more ascent on the ladder to overall parity. The potential for such an approach to produce viable results locally and generally may not have been very great. It was superior, however, to the positive potential in the demand actually made on the Soviets to combine tactical restraint with strategic retreat from the area as evidence of their good faith.

The failure to offer a meaningful test for the long term was obscured in the event by the brief high drama of an overadvertised confrontation. This had two immediate consequences. One was the proliferation of less pertinent and conclusive tests within the United States, such as the Jewish emigration issue. This jeopardized détente without really probing it. Another consequence was continuing underhanded competition with the Soviet Union over the peace issue in the Middle East. It did not equip the United States with the reservoir of domestic support that a previously demonstrated Soviet intractability would have created. Instead, the ensuing events weakened the domestic stamina in America by conjuring up the mirage of a diplomatic victory at the end of one more plane trip to be realized without the costs of either conflict or concert with the Soviet Union. As the mirage faded, the collapse of unreal hopes intensified the noxious interplay between Kissinger's exceptionally free diplomatic hand, having ever less to grasp at, and the oppositional (including congressional) free-for-all that was unlikely to generate new opportunities and approaches either by itself or in the belatedly sought executive-legislative partnership.

Great or small, apparent or real, the inadequacies in relations with the greater powers were supplemented by questionable procedures in the peacemaking strategies among lesser-power contestants. By eschewing both conflict and concert with the Communist great powers on specific issues, Kissinger confined his peacemaking diplomacy to the unproductive middle ground of low-level competition and limited cooperation for avoiding the ultimate confrontation. This kind of relations with the great powers helped paralyze the groping for a comparable middle ground in both Southeast Asia and the Middle East: a middle ground, that is, between peace based on the hegemonial preponderance of one contestant (North Vietnam, as a territorial power, and Israel), circumscribed mainly from the outside, and peace based on the resolute suppression or indefinite denial of the local revolutionary force seeking the total destruction of the adversary (Hanoi and the radical Arab-Palestinian wing as revolutionary agents). It was acceptable to treat North Vietnam as having the dual identity of conventional power and revolutionary force for the purposes of the different extreme solutions, just as it was to make Israel apparently the beneficiary under both. It was or ought to have been within the means of practical policy to implement the distinction in the first case and nuance the advantages accruing to one party in the second. What may have been more difficult for practical policy was to achieve results if the polcy was not equipped to contemplate and carry out at least one of the extreme solutions. And it may have been virtually impossible to conduct effective policy for either area without reference to the other area and to both of the Communist great powers.

There was little public evidence to show that Kissinger's peacemaking diplomacy conformed to either of the requirements that would assimilate it to "Bismarckian" statecraft.[1] Immediately following the military cease-fire in Vietnam, American statecraft made no perceptible effort to turn the briefly fluid situation toward a more substantial political settlement. Instead, the peacemaker seemed first to indulge his battle fatigue and then to seek easier and fresher laurels in the Middle East in apparent oblivion of Southeast Asia—until the prospect of a hostile military breakthrough in Indochina and a diplomatic stalemate in the Middle East would again redirect attention, if only for the purposes of recriminations between the two branches of government.

[1] See pp. 53ff.

Whatever setbacks were to be registered in both regions, they were the reverse of the initial *éclat* of Kissinger's two-track approach to peacemaking. The first track led Kissinger to concentrate his prime effort at defusing the military situation at its most explosive level. This meant removing American active participation in Indochina and, in the Middle East, eliminating the possibility that the interpenetration of Arab and Israeli troops might reignite both local conflict and superpower confrontation in short order. It also meant, however, not least in the Middle East, removing the pressure that an "untenable" military situation was susceptible of exerting on the "intractable" political issues toward their substantive resolution. Once he had relieved the second, or political, track Kissinger tended to leave the peacemaking process to accommodation among gradually evolving local forces: wholly in Indochina and with only mediatory American participation in the Middle East. The method was inherently conservative in its distrust of mechanical social engineering. Its practitioner's confidence is with the healing qualities of progressive evolution in conditions of relative repose. As such, the method is also wholly at variance with both the Communist method and with the classic statecraft of the age preceding total wars. Both treat military and diplomatic operations as inseparable in action and in time. It is not enough for a military flare-up to provide an opening for the peacemaker by dissolving previously frozen attitudes, an advantage which Kissinger could readily appreciate when the course and outcome of the October war had presented him with a previously unequaled opportunity; unless attitudes are to congeal again, the iron of war has to be hammered into shapes of peace while it is still incandescent —the leverage used while it is in being.

Kissinger's approach had an initial success in Vietnam, in part because the Soviet Union cooperated with it. It slowed down into an early standstill or only minor progress in the Middle East, also—but not only—because the Soviet Union worked against it with comparable discretion. The last stages of the American disengagement in Indochina were attended by an orchestration of military and diplomatic activity that was aimed at the Communist great powers at least as much as at Hanoi. A comparable orchestration of diplomatic and military means and measures was harder to come by in the Middle Eastern peacemaking after the precipitate cease-fire and the improvident military disengagement of the local belligerents, apart from the time-honored elementary device of supplying arms or withholding them from Israel. The situation was basically different, and so were the available means of pressure and inducement. In the Middle East, it has been an ally or dependent of the United States, Israel, which has held the expansive position in the conflict, not the North Vietnamese adversary. Hence, the military pressure via punishment (blockade and bombing) had to be replaced by pressure through actual or implicitly threatened denials (of arms). The relatively weaker coercive leverage in the Middle East actually available could be offset by the greater potency of inducements. These included, among other things, economic aid to Israel for oil purchases from Iran (to replace supplies from the militarily held Egyptian oil fields if and when evacuated). In both volume and reliability, aid to Israel exceeded both the U.S. aid pledges to Egypt and the promises of economic reconstruction aid to Hanoi. Also, there was less need or room for seeking to gain the cooperation of the immediately critical Communist great power, the Soviet Union, in exerting pressure on Israel to yield positions than had been the case with Hanoi. Conversely, the necessity for deterring a Soviet counteraction (in Syria and with the Palestinian Liberation Organization) promised to be greater if the United States pushed too hard on its basic leverage: in Southeast Asia the leverage had been American "unilateral" air and naval operations against Hanoi and Haiphong within the privileged sanctuary constituted by Soviet forbearance; in the Middle East the leverage consisted of the privileged U.S. diplomatic access to local parties permitting unilateral mediation and conciliation. The American advantage was increasingly challenged by the Soviets, as mediatory diplomacy persisted while the material benefits of détente that had been held out as an inducement for tolerance or better in Southeast Asia were losing their compensatory potency.

Military immunity for the United States in Southeast Asia had been largely due to China's prior rebound from the Soviet Union into militant independence and defensive insecurity vis-à-vis the erstwhile ally and protector in the Korean war. Similarly, the diplomatic opportunities of Kissinger's mediatory diplomacy in the Middle East were principally due to Egypt's rebound from the

Soviet ally and protector in the two preceding rounds of conflict—
and, as such, were both dedicated to and contingent upon sufficiently speedy progress to insure avoidance of yet another round of
conflict. This was the unique and unprecedented "chance" of
American diplomacy in the Middle East. Just as Dean Acheson
could not have rearranged the relations of power and policy in
Asia before Mao's alliance with the Soviet Union ran its frustrating
course, so John Foster Dulles and his successors before Kissinger
could do little or nothing in the Middle East before Nasserite
Egypt traversed a parallel itinerary. The remaining and possibly
unsurmountable obstacle was the substitution of Sadat Egypt's
economic dependence on conservative and oil-rich Arab Powers
for Nasser's claim to political dominance over radical Arab forces.
Both acted as a restraint on a unilateral Egyptian accommodation
with Israel that would remove in one form or another the free use
of the Egyptian armed forces from the Middle Eastern war-peace
equation. Egypt's new developmental domesticism was offset in its
positive effect on peacemaking by fear of Arab reprisals couched
in terms of pan-Arab solidarity. This was broadly equivalent in the
negative effect on settlement with the inhibition implicit in North
Vietnam's commitment to local or regional hegemony, couched in
terms of Marxist-Leninist ideology. It was doubtful that either of
the obstacles could be overcome by adjustments among local
forces alone, or by American efforts occurring outside a larger
great-power context.

III

The public appreciation of Kissinger's conservative system has
come to depend too much on his performance as regional peacemaker. The drama of obstinate conciliation efforts overshadowed
the paradoxes and contradictions in the decisive great-power dimension of the design. Being immediately centered in the U.S.-
Soviet détente, the design was contingent for long-term consolidation and extension on a continuing concurrence of the underlying
theses with major existential trends. Basically, the conservative
design was recommended by its apparent fit with the structure of
the contemporary international system. Likewise basically, it could
be challenged on the basis of its questionable fit with the develop-

mental stage of the United States as a major power, after discounting as only temporary the depressed psychopolitical state of the domestic polity and its economy. Deriving from the basic query and related to it are questions concerning the conservative design's standing with respect to the critical interplay between the mechanical (interactive) and organic (developmental-evolutionary) dimensions in international politics as well as to the critical relation between a specific strategy or strategies and the underlying doctrine or philosophy—or philosophies. The central question is whether the United States has indeed already become a relatively declining power in material and psychological capacity, needful of prudential nursing internationally, and whether the conservative design is not such as to initiate that decline (if it had not set in already) or aggravate and deepen it (if it had).

The central question overshadows the issue of compatibility between the long-range objectives which the two superpowers have been seeking to secure by détente. Since Kissinger's policy of appeasement unfolded not so much from strength as from an initially superior position, it unavoidably involved concessions if, as may be safely assumed, the minimum "constructive" objective of the Soviet Union was overall parity. The American concessions could be more or less graduated and more or less compensated for and, consequently, the process of "equalization" be more or less controlled or controllable from a position of leadership in equilibrium politics. The task was beset by paradoxes, however. For one, if a gradual process of reciprocal accommodation and, up to a point, assimilation could unfold only over a very long term, the initial U.S. assets readily available for compensation were of a kind to be quickly exhausted. And for another, while the concessionary process was beset by limits on particular concessions, its very dynamic was such that it threatened to prematurely upset the psychopolitical—even if not the material—balance between the two parties to the disadvantage of the United States. On the first score, the policy of appeasement with the Soviet Union and to a degree also with China could be seen as one of gradually integrating the two Communist powers into the international system by virtue of legitimizing concessions of a formal nature, essentially relating to status, more or less in exchange for "good behavior." Such formal concessions can be broadly construed to encompass nuclear standing along with a role in international organization, privileged consultations, or conspicuous exchanges of high-level diplomatic courtesies such as summits, state visits, and the like. It is in the nature of such formal concessions, however, that their symbolic significance is soon used up. Their supply is thus limited, and once made, they can be withdrawn with difficulty, if at all. This fact will quickly transfer the burden of the accommodation policy to more specific and material concessions.

In the U.S.-Soviet relations, both Kissinger's basic strategy (to conserve essential U.S. assets pending consolidation of and by détente) and the static nature of U.S. relations with both principal allies and, following "normalization," with China imposed definite limits on such concessions. Concessions from a "superior" to an "inferior" power can continue indefinitely only if the former manages an indefinite generation of ever new assets of its own from which to allocate a steady or growing share to the "rising" power. To do this has not been within U.S. capacity. In any other situation, concessionary diplomacy, if it is not to be self-liquidating, is interdependent with constellating diplomacy. That is, concessions can be made with relative impunity if they are distributed between powers that are—or can be—counterpoised in reciprocal rivalry and are, consequently, potentially neutralized in their depressing effect on the power making the concession (e.g., concessions to the Soviet Union in the Middle East and to China in Southeast Asia); if they bear on assets that have become irrelevant or even counterproductive in the new constellation (e.g., degrees of alliance integration or force-levels in a more complex equilibrium situation); or, finally, if they do not so much cancel themselves out as they are compensated for by new assets that are automatically or spontaneously generated by the new constellation—in the form of additional access or diplomatic options, reduced hostility with one power amounting to additional leverage over another, and more flexibility in general. Any such widening of scope for concessions to the Soviet Union, notably in matters with conventional politico-strategic or geopolitical significance, required shifting priority from consolidating two-power détente to consolidating a three-to-four power equilibrium situation. The absence of such effort meant that the concessionary spectrum would or could be activated mainly or only at its symbolic and material (economic and technological) extremes, while being nearly paralyzed at the critical middle of the range involving strategically significant political behavior, objectives, and values.

The precarious state of things was provisionally sustainable as long as the economic-technological interests of the Soviet Union in détente seemed susceptible of being satisfied. But difficulties could not but arise as soon as internal opposition to technological transfers and commercial credits in the United States was either aroused or amplified by developments which made the symbolic concessions controversial and the near-paralyzed sector of politico-strategic issues perversely explosive. If the first was due to doubts about the relationship of the SALT agreements to nuclear "sufficiency" (if not "superiority"), the second was due to the substitution of illegitimate extraneous tests of Soviet détente-mindedness for insufficient or nonexistent authoritative tests. Such developments imparted politically significant salience to doubts of experts (nourished by reexaminations of the post–World War I experience) about the utility of transferring technological strength to the Soviet Union in isolation from broader issues—such as liberalization in politico-economic policies and, possibly, uses and abuses of the new economic and strategic dimensions of the oceans. Political considerations and constraints were reinforced when even specific economic *quid pro quos* were not sufficiently attractive to vindicate an apolitical approach to détente through many-faceted functional agreements. And practically significant disparities in the basic operational modes of the two economic systems surfaced as *the* critical hurdle when the earlier impediment to more active exchanges had faded with the discarding of concern over comparative growth rates between the two superpowers in favor of a new and more pressing concern over the possibility of continuing economic growth at all, in separation from the ideological context, in the United States or in the industrial sector of the world economy as a whole (marginally including the Soviet Union itself). Finally, and perhaps decisively, the mineral-rich Soviet Union has been radically improving its balance of trade with the West, and with Western Europe in particular. This has enabled it to cover many of its technological needs independently of détente-related American credits.

In the political realm even more and earlier than in the economic one, the détente policy impinged critically upon America's relations with major allies, notably in Western Europe but also in Asia (Japan). The problems revolved around the two unequally and asymmetrically ·interdependent relationships between the United States and the allies and between the American policy of détente with the Soviet Union and continuing control over the allies. In the key domain of strategic security, the first and more basic interdependence has been sufficient, and sufficiently unequal, to permit the United States to exert independent initiatives vis-à-vis third powers and effective persuasion vis-à-vis the allies themselves. The interdependence has been neither sufficient nor sufficiently or one-sidedly unequal in respect to all material factors and policy options, however, to prevent the allies from reacting with lower-level initiatives of their own and either resisting or retaliating against American efforts at persuasion. The result was a situation which made the U.S.-Soviet détente possible and relatively easy to initiate while making its longer-term course precarious and some of its side-effects unpredictable.

While the fact of U.S.-allied interdependence reflected fundamental conditions and interests, its specific manifestations were also increasingly a function of the second interdependent relationship, that between détente and control. In Kissinger's conservative design, continuing control over the principal allies in Europe was the precondition of a U.S.-managed détente in the military-strategic area (SALT; negotiations over force reductions in Europe) as well as in the geopolitical area (the German problem, also as related to Eastern Europe and to the issues involved in all-European "security" and "cooperation"). This explained the official American displeasure over independent West German initiatives in *Ostpolitik* in the earlier Nixon-Kissinger phase, however strikingly these initiatives may have implemented the broad goals of détente. Continued control over allies had the advantage of insuring a relatively "cheap" détente: i.e., control insured a minimum of disruption in pre-détente conditions and thus a minimum of changes of advantage to the Soviet Union. Ideally, détente itself would in turn facilitate continuing control over the allies at less cost than before. Basically, the quite substantial continuing U.S. control over inter-allied relations insured that the American side in the balance of power with the Soviet Union would not promptly decline below an acceptable level as a result of détente. Conversely, détente with the Soviet Union would create a new U.S.-European balance of interests in the alliance, permitting the United States to perpetuate control in the form of alliance leadership on more economical terms than previously. This would happen as the détente codified the lowered risk of war in Europe. Since a war in Europe would be militarily the responsibility of the United States itself both in the first place and in the last resort, the virtual disappearance of the prospect of war would enable the United States to match the European posture of relative detachment on this subject, a posture originally introduced by French diplomacy under de Gaulle. Deterrence and defense functions would be disjoined in effect as factors in the inter-allied balance of concerns and, consequently, individual performances and reciprocal concessions.

A mere commitment to détente sufficed to set the stage for U.S. self-assertion on the economic issues in 1971; the unfolding of détente permitted the continuance of a tough American stand on the institutional issues in 1973 and 1974. The first linked American production of security with European (and world) consumption of American export goods. Residual insecurity was just sufficient to insure European abidance by the arbitrament implicit in the U.S. leverage; actual security was sufficient to make the leverage a practically usable one for the United States. The second issue, that of the U.S. role in intra-European consultations, was merged to U.S. advantage with the revival of insecurity in a new, economic garb in connection with the energy crisis and its initial impact on the West European economies. Once the Soviet Union "chose" the United States over Western Europe (be it de Gaulle's France, West Germany, or a Franco-German combine) as the preferred partner in détente, Soviet political intrigue in Western Europe aimed at American presence and influence was likely to be minimized, though not eliminated. But the same choice did not automatically reduce incentives to politically motivated Soviet economic intrigue—e.g., in the Middle East on oil. This fact insured that any economy in the outlays incurred in upholding the U.S. preponderance in Western Europe, due to declining politico-military strains in the atmosphere of détente, would not be automatically matched by an increase leeway for the Western Europeans, due to their rising collective economic power. As a matter of fact, insofar as the oil crisis was partially traceable to the diminished capacity of U.S. policymakers to wield political deterrence vis-à-vis the OPEC countries from the post-Vietnam stance, of which détente was a major aspect, the consequences of détente for U.S. influence were self-equilibrating. They would be such as long as any diminution of the threat of a Soviet hegemony was canceled out by a new threat. The threat from an (Arab) oil-producer hegemony was sufficient to shore up, for the time being, the eroding bases of the political American hegemony in Western Europe (and, comparably, Japan), and it permitted hard bargaining over the cost of American support for the allies against the newly structured aggregate threat.

Normally and logically, any decline in the Soviet threat would be attended by a marked reduction of U.S. control in Western Europe. In actuality, the scope of such reduction has been contained so far while the actual or henceforth feasible reduction of effective costs incurred by the United States in maintaining control via its defense and support role exceeded any actual or necessary reduction in that control. Since the United States depended on an American presence in Western Europe (and Japan) for an effective détente policy with the Soviets more palpably than the continuance of essential American influence among principal allies was a function of the détente itself and its consequences, the relationship between détente and control has been one of unequal interdependence. The related fact—the United States "needing" Western Europe for immediate purposes of global policy more than Western Europe needed the United States for immediate security—engendered a potential for reversing the other, more significant and original, inequality—in the interdependence between Western Europe and the U.S. themselves—to Europe's advantage. If the reversal was not implemented in an effective restructuring of relations, this was due to the collective incapacity of the West Europeans as well as to the both crude and subtle American reinforcements of that incapacity. American diplomacy was able to thwart, in effect, the development of a formal or institutional European "identity" by way of a consultative mechanism that would reduce American capacity for interposition in early stages of intra-European consultations. And the essential *status quo* was reconfirmed, at least temporarily, by the new opportunities opened up for American leadership by the material implications of the oil crisis. This was the concrete meaning of the earlier contention[2] that Kissinger hectored the Europeans over their best efforts while shielding them from the worst emergencies.

The resulting situation, while favorable to immediate American objectives, was not necessarily equally favorable to the success of the détente policy in the longer run. Initially, the working of the American-European relationship under the impact of U.S. initiatives and pressures facilitated détente by permitting agreements with the Soviet Union in such areas as nuclear stability and all-European security and cooperation, on the basis of not always wholly matched Western concessions and Soviet gains—either "new" or legitimated "old." Beyond that, a continuing development of détente was liable to suffer, without eliminating the possibility that the Soviets would realize nonetheless one of their possible objectives of détente: the erosion of U.S.-European (as well as Japanese) ties and thus erosion of "Western" strength. One major reason was that the basically unreformed interallied relationship inhibited, along with Western European "independence," effective coordination of policies within the alliance. Continuing U.S. involvement and controls impeded intra-European coordination both directly—by feeding into Franco-German-British differences—and indirectly—by diminishing the incentive for independent joint European adaptation to both continuing problems (defense) and emergent critical problems (oil). Nor was this all. If the *fact* of continuing U.S. protection, as an aspect of control and its basis, has impeded the development of a political European identity that would counteract economically motivated disunities within Western Europe, the diminished *need* for protection (due to détente) has reduced political unity between Western Europe and the United States as a corrective to growing economic differences between them. Moreover, any and all European suspicions of the United States placing détente with the Soviet Union above trans-Atlantic political relations further impeded confidence and cooperation among the allies, while official Americans looked with mixed feelings on the relatively faster-growing economic relations of Western Europe with Communist Europe.

[2] See p. 68.

81

Inadequate interallied coordination could have at any time the immediate consequence of impeding explicit bargaining with the Soviet Union over reciprocal concessions while facilitating uncompensated *de facto* Soviet intrusions and keeping open the possibility and temptation for the allies to outbid one another in the pursuit of special economic and, eventually, also political arrangements with the Soviets in the longer run. The standing danger along these lines was for U.S.-Soviet détente to degenerate into competitive *détentisme* among the Western allies, and to do so at a time and stage when the consequent potential for a division of political or diplomatic labor among the allies would no longer have the compensating advantages that had been inherent in the early unilateral initiatives in favor of "relaxing" cold-war tensions. A different—and possibly more immediately damaging—set of consequences attached to the combination of deficiencies, in European "independence" and interallied coordination, with an excess, i.e., in the outsiders' tendency to identify Western Europe with the United States none the less. The immediate victim was concessionary diplomacy and its indispensable component, coercive diplomacy. It was harder for the United States to make strategic-political concessions to the Soviet Union, say in the Middle East, without further alienating China by evidence of superpower collusion if there was no "independent" Europe that could compensate for the resulting slack in (U.S.) pressure on the Soviet Union by coordinating action with China on Eastern Europe, if not Southeast Asia, in the last resort. So much has been noted already. But it was likewise difficult to make concessions in the absence of a demonstrable ready capacity for confrontational diplomacy. The capacity was limited as long as a Western Europe that was being identified with the United States without being consulted had every reason to deny cooperation in U.S. military deployments into the Middle East, for instance, in order to protect itself from economic and other reprisals at Arab hands. A Western Europe without effective and in part independent self-defense capacity has remained, despite détente, a Soviet hostage for U.S. good behavior in the last resort. A politically disunited and dispirited Western Europe, preoccupied with trade and shrinking from every tremor liable to upset its delicate economies, was a brake on the coercive aspects of effective U.S. action also in relation to economically strong and potentially retaliatory powers such as the Middle Eastern oil-producers.

Weak in the traditional forms of power and weaker still in traditional readiness to use available power, the Western Europeans inclined increasingly to claim for themselves the right to a certain opportunism as the last resort and compensatory privilege of those of inferior status. It was the questionably correct but understandable belief behind that attitude, on the strength of the new post–de Gaulle Europe's increasingly Japan-like economic preoccupations over against the primarily or ultimately political ones of nearly everybody else, that the "old" issues of political independence versus interdependence within the Atlantic community were becoming obsolete also as the threat of an oil-based Arab economic hegemony over Western Europe was being converted into an Euro-Arab economic community on the basis of a complementarity that would usefully supplement the differently asymmetrical one with large parts of Africa. Like preceding administrations, the Nixon administration and its successor countered suggestions of U.S. co-responsibility for this state of things with the claim that the Europeans (and the Japanese) would not have it otherwise, despite American coaxing of the Europeans, if not of the Japanese, to move toward greater self-reliance also in defense and related matters. Yet even if American exhortations were sincere (which must, beyond a certain point, be questioned on grounds of incompatibility with the global détente design), a question would still remain. The question is whether a vital supplement to the exhortation to seize possibilities for enlarged independence is not exposure to the necessity to do so; whether structurally conditioned immobilism must not or ought not be overcome by strategically encompassed mobilization.

Mobilizing Western Europe politically required the United States to manipulate constellations. This would differ from either managing détente by keeping Western Europe dependent or, even, from steering Western Europe toward greater self-dependence or complementarity with the United States as an alternative to détente or a priority over it. It is unlikely that even the best will on the part of American policymakers could restructure U.S.-European relations in a straight line of a "step-by-step" cumulative process, or as a matter of interaction confined to the two parties, without the extraneous stimulant of a global re-constellation involving third powers. Only a new world setting, involving at the very least the even activation of both of the Communist great powers, could generate sufficient incentives for the Europeans to act—and sufficient risks from not acting—to inspire efforts to fit a politically unified Western Europe into the new global configuration as an "equal" party. The new situation would have to be one in which the United States had patent grounds for discounting its stake in Western Europe and would be, therefore, both free to relax and, in order to realize the utmost potential of the new constellation, motivated to relax controls in Western Europe that had been perpetuated in order to avoid prematurely losing the Western European asset in the absence of an effective Chinese or other counterpoise to the Soviet Union. The new situation would also have to be such as to encourage the Western Europeans to cease clinging to the United States for fear of seeing it go all the way to an American-Soviet global condominium, further downgrading Western Europe's significance if not its security. If, in a four-power setting, an independent Western Europe would be valuable to China as a potential "ally" in relations with both the United States and the Soviet Union, and China would be a valued supplemental counterweight against the Soviet Union for Western Europe, the Soviet Union would be valuable to Western Europe—if not as either an ally or counterpoise against the United States, then as an alternative source of possible easements. Such easements could occur, for instance, if the far-reaching Euro-Soviet community of political views on the Arab-Israeli relationship were translated into Soviet aid in relieving pressures from the oil front directly or by way of influence in the Middle East indirectly.

In the past, the insufficient French power base of de Gaulle's diplomacy precluded it from creating from within Western Europe the opportunity for regional independence by way of de-ideologized relations with both the Soviet Union and, as an inducement to the Soviets to take de Gaulle seriously, Maoist China. Kissinger's triangular diplomacy preempted the initiative for the United States without developing the de Gaulle line from a position of superior American strength far enough to consummate the line's intended long-term effect in Europe. American diplomacy did little to "force" Western Europe, by exposing it to global multilateralization, to assume the kind of independent posture into which it would not "follow" de Gaulle's exhortations. Quite to the contrary, the "year of Europe" Kissinger style nearly coincided with the end of an active China policy; and Kissinger's approach to interallied relations hewed closer to the Kennedyite "great design" for an unequal Atlantic partnership than to the Gaullist grand strategy for an equalized global de-polarization. Imitation of the Gaullist diplomatic procedure went with the perversion of its purpose: normalization with Peking, not to start consummating Europe's military liberation by the United States in World War II with its diplomatic liberation from the United States, but only to liberate American statecraft from the war in Vietnam and thus free it for the reimposition of "hegemony" in the Atlantic theater.

The situation has been in many respects similar as regards the other principal U.S. ally, Japan. Her strategic-diplomatic activation entailed reducing both the regional (Far Eastern) ramifications and the bilateral intimacy of the U.S.-Japanese security treaty. It could most usefully only follow the activation of Western Europe (or, in the absence thereof, West Germany?). The European preliminary would not only routinize the new multipolar international politics, moderating thus the adverse impact of a new Japanese activism among the lesser powers of Asia. A delay would also permit the internal Japanese political system to begin adjusting to the eventual relaxing of an exclusive American connection. On balance, that connection has been internally stabilizing for Japan and has become provisionally reassuring for both the Soviet Union and China, since it spared Japan premature choices between a (spontaneously?) pro-China and an (enforced?) pro-Soviet orientation in the free-wheeling four-power equilibrium politics in Asia that would ensue upon the loosening of the U.S.-Japanese ties. In due course, however, Japan's gradual advance toward greater self-reliance for defense and independence in high policy was, again on balance, a useful and even necessary element in multipolar equilibrium politics. The basic or ultimate reason lies in the probability that greater Japanese "independence" would serve (next to China's "parity") as an additional disincentive to Soviet-Chinese recoalescence, inasmuch as one or both of the Communist powers would rightly perceive such fusion as one likely to drive Japan back into the arms of the United States. Should Sino-Soviet recoalescence take place nonetheless, a previously activated Japan would be all the more valuable as a more effective counterpoise to the restored "bloc" in Asia. The obverse possibility, that an activation of China with U.S. assistance would frighten Japan and drive her into the arms of the Soviet Union, has not been a serious one in view of Japan's at worst ambivalent attitude to China and the continuance—or even reinforcement—of both American and Soviet counterpoise to China in a multipolar situation. To judge otherwise was to postulate the necessity of keeping on desultory diplomatic terms with China and entertaining close relations with only the Soviets in order to minimize Japan's recoil to the Soviet Union and Soviet receptivity to Japan's advances, or outright wooing of Japan, in competition with the United States. In such a view, the U.S. would become the captive of U.S.-Soviet détente in Asia even while the basis for equal benefits from détente was in danger of deteriorating in Europe.

Even as it was intended to minimize other risks, Kissinger's conservative design harbored an unavoidable major one. It was the risk that delaying devolution in both Europe and Asia until détente had consolidated U.S.-Soviet relations would remove all the other preconditions for such devolution. That is to say, delays could alienate China into either revolutionary Third-World politics or recoalescence with the Soviet Union, either of which would more or less critically compound the adverse shifts in power and influence already occurring in Asia. And delays did not guarantee the projected timetable against either incremental or genuinely revolutionary politico-economic transformation in a dispirited Western Europe already beset by adverse developments of one kind or another on its extreme flanks and extremities (Portugal as well as her one-time protector, Great Britain; Italy as well as again-embattled Greece and Turkey). Any further deterioration would annihilate the possibility of the Western Europeans leaving the American "hegemony" for independence as a collective entity—rather than falling individually under a different hegemony—even when finally invited to do so. If, however, American-Soviet détente were to culminate in the dissolution of Western Europe rather than in the dissolution of U.S.-European "interdependence" in its present forms (perhaps conjointly with a resolution of the Sino-Soviet conflict), it would have exacted also the price of a decline in the

U.S. position relative to the Soviet Union, quite apart from what happened in the United States itself in the process. In such conditions, competitive *détentisme* in the West would be liable to gather speed on all fronts and be "won" by West Germany over France in the first round and over the United States itself in the second. The resulting cumulative decline would be neutralized only by an unimpeded unfolding of competitive decadence[3] encompassing also the Soviet Union—a form of "parity" that was unlikely to prevail over one-sidedly favorable trends in the world at large.

In Kissinger's Metternichian system, America's "presiding power" in Western Europe has been the equivalent of Austria's in post-Napoleonic Germany. The older system was sustained by Russia's support for Austrian constraints on revolution; the more recent one has come to be (provisionally?) favored by the Soviet Union as constituting a constraint on Germany's politico-military resurgence. Both the Austrian and the American supremacies were, moreover, sustained by the reluctance of the German and the European states, respectively, to receive more stringent unity at the hands of the most dynamic one among them: from Prussia in Germany and, in Western Europe, from diplomatically dynamic France in the Gaullist phase and, possibly, from economically dynamic West Germany in the future. There were important differences, though. As long as it is not replaced by another outside power, the United States depends on direct presence or dominance in Western Europe for its position as a world power less than Austria needed her role in Germany to be a European power of the first rank. Consequently, outside NATO, the United States has been able to exercise influence in the Western European institutions less directly than Austria did in the organs of the Germanic Confederation. The United States was, moreover, in principle able to relax such controls still further without detriment to its essential interests. In the longer view, it was in the positive American interest to do so, if only to lessen the possibility that a virtually depoliticized Western Europe be wholly permeated by narrowly economic values at the popular level and by related policy criteria at the élite levels. The longer could existing tendencies in that direction continue, the greater was the prospect that Europe would not be even-

---

[3] The phrase "competitive decadence" is Pierre Hassner's.

tually unified from within Western Europe, in mere self-differentiation from America. Instead, a socially or morally rudderless Western Europe—possibly swayed by its German microcosm—might one day respond to the battle cry of historic European identity and unity raised by peaceful means, if in outright opposition to the United States, by its more primitive counterpart in the East. In a similar manner, somewhat as contemporary Vietnam, ancient Egypt was unified from the more primitive upper Nile and not from the commercialized cities of the delta; Germany from traditional Prussia and not from the Rhenish parts; and Italy from Piedmont and not from either Venice or Rome.

IV

In the event of any adverse development of whatever specific kind, a strategy of deferred gradualism—i.e., step-by-step devolution only following the initial détente phase—might well prove to have been only a prescription for the full eventual unfolding of the catastrophic strain that is implicit in at least one strand of Kissinger's own "philosophy of history." A full relationship between diplomatic strategy and political philosophy involves the interplay and relative ordering of the mechanical and the organic aspects of politics, including international politics, within both strategy and philosophy. The "mechanical" dimension involves interaction and manipulations of readily available or accessible forces; the "organic" one comprises the only marginally manageable development of the tangible and intangible elements of power. The essence of the first is counterpoising through checks and balances in diplomatic strategy; of the second, the juxtaposition of growth and decline dynamics in an international system. If the first entails deliberately fostered competition over the distribution of widely coveted identical stakes, the second involves a given differentiation among states at different stages of development.

The early Nixon-Kissinger diplomacy drew on the interplay when it initially surfaced the previously transpired organic changes in the principal great powers by manipulating Sino-Soviet differences for a specific purpose. The subsequent conservative design of Kissinger's, as so far discussed, failed to persevere in the attempt to manipulatively promote an unfolding of the desired or desirable growth-decline factors and trends. That is to say, the détente policy with the Soviet Union was not integrated into a devolutionary policy. Such policy would aim at instigating the diffusion of other than Soviet power and role so as to create the conditions for containing an intemperate or asymmetric growth of Soviet or Soviet-cum-allied power. In failing to promote a sustained active participation by China in international diplomacy, and the consequent activation of Western Europe (and Japan) within the restructured international system, the conservative design threatened to demote the Western side of the U.S.-Soviet balance. As part of the relative decline, Western Europe would decay into a combination of *attentisme*[4] (vis-à-vis the "limited" U.S.-Soviet competition and its outcome) and "alibism" (vis-à-vis raw-material producers in the Third World antagonized by U.S. policies as part of that competition); and the wearied United States would subside into a combination of economic autarky and, as part of it, political imperialism within a narrowed scope. The consequently deranged relations between the "West" and the Third World would reflect the failure of a policy which, in addition to mismanaging relations among the actual and potential great powers, misapplied the mechanical-organic dimension also relative to the middle and small powers both intra- and inter-regionally in immediately war-torn or only latently crisis-ridden areas; a policy which made no sustained and visible effort either to stimulate the rise of core-powers capable of exercising moderate hegemony or to safeguard local and extra-regional capacity for reactive containing response to unrestrainedly domineering core-powers; and a policy which failed to evolve, as part of such an effort, a great-power superstructure for the intra- and inter-regionally balanced hierarchies by combining *ad hoc* concert and conflict/confrontation in one strategy. Some such procedure was necessary to help evolve rudimentary balance-of-power systems as preliminaries to workable regional associations for order and development.

In the absence of a sustained strategic effort also in the Third World, the conservative design—combining U.S.-Soviet détente

---

[4] A derivative from *attendre* (wait), this word was coined for the wartime policy of Vichy while the outcome of the Axis-United Nations contest appeared uncertain.

with the retention of most pre-détente American assets—was liable to degenerate into drift and erosion from a base already weakened in the essential sector of allied and adversary great powers. Pending clarification of its structural objectives, the limitations of Kissinger's statecraft for the Third World were manifest mainly in its procedure. The apparent failure to link within a policy two or more conflicts or issues involving greater and lesser powers in the different regions of the Third World—and, when occasion permitted or erosion of leverages in the Third World required, also in Europe—produced a generalized "shuttle diplomacy" characterized by a rushing from one isolated issue or conflict to another. Dealing with issues separately and pragmatically on their "merits" may be innate to American foreign policy making. The procedure was also the consequence of Kissinger's own more recent failure to activate the great-power handles on local situations within a system-wide diplomacy as the antithesis of his shuttle diplomacy. Concurrently, the absence of a systematic devolution strategy led to an uncompensated localized erosion of U.S. positions—e.g., the commitment to a timed extrusion of American forces from Thailand by a succession of weak coalition governments in separation from, and in the absence of, any perceptible U.S. role in restructuring the wider regional balance of power as it related to both China and Indochina.

Such forms of dubiously masterful inactivity in a key Third-World area (Asia) complemented a strategically unsupported mediatory activism for peaceful change in another area (the Middle East) and the masterly inhibition of systemic change in yet another segment of the international system (Western Europe). All could be vindicated only in a long retrospect by the then demonstrable "rightness" of either the tactical precepts at one extreme or the basic doctrinal-philosophical premise on another. Both precept and premise are of a peculiar conservative kind. The tactical precept was to insulate or ignore the remainder of the overall environment if one was to effectively modify, or concentrate upon, the most critical or pressing sector at any one time. This meant concentrating on détente while keeping Western Europe constant, and on the Middle East while ignoring Southeast Asia. The tactic is one which economizes on energy: both the system-wide energy that would be released by a more comprehensive strategy and the personal, physical, and intellectual energy to be expended by the strategist himself. The more routine approach will work only if and as long as the tactically decisive conditions are exceptionally favorable, as they appeared to be for a time in the Middle East in the diplomatic sector and were up to a point in Europe as a spillover from the Middle Eastern derangements in the economic sector; it will be successful on a wider basis in the longer run only if the more fundamental structural and psychological factors prove to have been likewise propitious. This will require the existential trends to coincide with—and thus support—the theses underlying the tactics which, in such a favorable case, attain the more exalted status of strategy.

Let it be supposed that Kissinger's conservative design was faulty along the so-far suggested or similar lines in "normal" or "neutral" conditions and in some degree at least. To that same extent it would depend for success on uniquely favorable conditions, and for rightness on a controlling political philosophy or doctrine which correctly postulated such unique conditions. Conversely, the internal structure of the philosophic doctrine might actually compound any defects in the diplomatic strategy. A critical defect in Kissinger's strategy would be misjudgments about the relation of détente to decay and thus about the fit between the conservative strategy and the developmental stages of the parties to détente.

The most striking aspect of Kissinger's philosophy was its explicit pessimism and implicit optimism. The duality had significant and potentially negative implications for the conservative design. In impromptu or off-the-record musings, Kissinger tended to be philosophically pessimistic about the West in general—and about Western Europe in particular. On "procedural" grounds, such pessimism concerned the capacity of the post-Vietnam United States for effective, specifically including conventional military, action; the capacity of Europe to produce governments that would be both efficacious and legitimate; and the capacity to arrive at effective decisions either in the United States (by routinized bureaucratic procedures or in executive-legislative interactions) or jointly with major allies (if Western Europe were to be allowed to preformulate decisions in initial separation from American interposition). On "substantive" grounds, pessimism centered on the vulnerability of individual European countries to communization, as an aspect of a generalized Western lack or loss of political, socio-economic, or moral resilience and resistance.

If Kissinger's pessimism concerning the West was even half-meant (or, alternatively, if its description here is only half-correct), then it presupposed a sort of "optimism" about trends in the rest of the world to qualify Kissinger's conservative design as an at all responsible one. To be "optimistic," assumptions with regard to the Communist great powers—the Soviet Union in the first place and in the shorter run and China secondarily over the longer term—would have to postulate evolution toward ever more "responsible" governments and "realistic" policies, even if avoiding the expectation of socio-political and ideological "convergence" at the foundations. In the more limited view, revolutionary policies and goals would yield to conventional goals identified with the national interest. Ideological commitments would be simultaneously eroded by the mutually reinforcing effects of increased domestic affluence and legitimized international influence, the first aided by the diffusion of Western technological assets and the resulting economic interdependence while the second was both facilitated and controlled by a likewise gradual diffusion of status-related prestige assets. The diffusion of material and immaterial values would stimulate the desired development as part of both functional interrelations and diplomatic transactions. It would thus be possible to contain the scope of demands for major changes in the critical balances of militarily-strategically or geopolitically defined positions of power within the limits set by a critical difference: the difference between a conservatively managed transformation of U.S. primacy into a new equilibrium and the historically more common transfer of international primacy from a declining state to a rising power and thus a new empire.

A matching optimism in relation to the Third World required belief that, concurrently with the reduction of the expansionist drives of the Communist great powers aimed at preempting previously U.S.-held positions, at least some Third-World countries would mature economically and politically, and that they would do so at a sufficient rate to have become responsive to the devolution of responsibilities for regional order when such a devolution had been made possible in terms of the relations among the great powers globally. At that deferred point, a mutually reinforcing subsidence of "revolution" in motivating behavior and growth of system-wide capacity for "devolution" as process and policy would insure that an effectively retrenching United States was replaced by a new, regionally deconcentrated international system and not by a new global imperial power and a spate of regionally imperialistic lesser powers.

This was the strongest case that could be made for a gradualist conservative design. It was difficult to see, however, how any such favorable developments could resist the adverse effects from the simultaneously posited Western weaknesses—even if these weaknesses were not augmented by the design itself. If this is true, it is still harder to justify a design or strategy which does little on the face of it to counteract in the realm of strategic activity the implications of the dualistic structure within the controlling philosophy. On the operative plane, it was questionable whether the American supply of material or economic and systemic or status assets would be sufficient—inherently and in terms of domestic political feasibility—to match the demands for redistribution by either the Communist great powers or the ambitious Third-World states that were implicit in the "optimistic" assumptions and, even more, in the relationship between the "optimistic" and the "pessimistic" assumptions. It was especially unlikely that the supply was sufficient in an essentially static diplomatic-strategic universe; one, that is, in which but few or limited changes in the constellation among the great powers alongside regional conflicts involving lesser states would be in evidence and could be depended upon to spontaneously replenish both the needs and the supply of one kind of asset, i.e., the prestige-political or systemic, and reduce the immediate significance or demand for the other kind of asset, i.e., the material-economic or specific.

V. BISMARCK VERSUS METTERNICH: BEYOND KISSINGER

The possibility of a contradiction between the hypothetically "optimistic" aspects of the conservative scenario and its "pessimistic" features raised questions, and gave justification to apprehensions, about the future. Meanwhile, the task for the present was to identify—and, if possible, weigh—the risks implicit in the by and large only tactically or routinely supported philosophic "wager," characteristic of the Metternichian design, in comparison with the risks adhering to the strategically enacted diplomatic "gambles," characteristic of the Bismarckian statecraft even at its most responsible and restrained.

I

There are at least two types of conservative political philosophy. They respond with different basic strategies to the duality between optimism and pessimism; and the strategies stress and exploit differently the opportunities and challenges engendered by the mechanical-organic interplay in international politics. Any conservative political philosophy will incline toward pessimism about so-called human nature, the likely or possible effect of deliberate human endeavor, and the likely and desirable effect of change on the preservation of dominant positions in a political system. Such similarity of outlook unifies conservative thought relative to its liberal or progressive opposite. Beyond it lies the fundamental difference between defiant and defeatist or despondent conservatism in both theory and practice. The first strand is identifiable with Bismarckian conservatism and the latter with the Metternichian (and, broadly, Kissinger's) outlook.

The defiant conservative operates from a still substantial residual strength; and he aims at conserving and consolidating essential positions by re-forming the political system. He will employ manipulative strategies to rearrange existing forces and release new supporting forces so as to contain or constrain the principal challenge to the established distribution of power by either a rival social class, a rival state, or an adverse internal or international coalition. Such was, parallel to international counterpoising aimed to preserve the newly won German position from a coalition around France's "revolutionary" revanchism, Bismarck's domestic politics. It was designed to fragment the political opposition to the continuing dominance of the traditional elements by parliamentary manipulation while both political (suffrage) and social (welfare) reforms were to create a conservatively controlled counterpoise to the ascendant industrial and intellectual middle class and, one step behind it, social democracy.

By contrast, the Metternichian type of domestic conservatism operates from an irreversibly waning strength; its basic political formula consists of dependent alliance of the traditional power (the "throne") with its classic supports, such as the Church (the "altar"), the army (the "sword"), and the socially privileged class or politically privileged ethnic group or groups. This supplements international dependence on a major conservative power or institution (a holy-alliance type of concert). The ideological camouflage for the Metternichian conservative's immediate dependence and deferral of defeat will be antirevolutionary "legitimacy," whereas the Bismarckian type would usurp the "revolutionary" mantle from the veritable radicals lurking in the wings.

The differences are fundamental. The defeatist conservative hazards only sporadic or peripheral management—or "nursing"— of forces and trends, in contrast to the defiant one's active or creative manipulation. And he sets up repose and refusal of change, punctuated by occasional repression, against reform for releasing new forces while they can still be controlled—or appear to be such. He would lean on what is, rather than seek to evolve leverages in order to contain what is coming. The difference between the two strands of conservatism is thus almost as great as the contrast between conservative reform and progressive liberal reform. The liberal would reform in order to improve and create a new type of society or political system; he would "finally" resolve the struggle over power in favor of an institutionalized allocation of the newly salient welfare values. On his part, the conservative would reform only in the sense of reshaping the balance of forces comprising established or residual forces, the potentially or actually resurgent or revolutionary, and the only remotely emerging. Where the liberal-progressive would transform the traditional system of power, the defiant conservative resists the transfer of dominant power. He bends every effort to sustain the essential elements of the old order while giving up on inessential appearances.

It is altogether possible for both types of conservative to be scheduled for ultimate defeat and for the conservative who was defiant in his middle age to end up in the despondent-defeatist category in his old age. But only while defiant is the conservative likely to leave a discernible imprint on the next-following provisional outcome while co-determining the contours and the length of the pathway from one socio-political order to another. This difference does not correspond to the basic attitudes of the two types of conservative, however. Paradoxically, it is the defiant conservative who is philosophically pessimistic all around; there is no worthwhile future unless the system is reshaped. By contrast, a perverse touch of optimism sustains the defeatist conservative; peripheral management just might suffice indefinitely if fundamental prudence about change is properly assorted with sporadic repression. Where the defiant conservative is, therefore, disposed to gamble on an effectively conserving outcome of risk-taking political or diplomatic strategies, the defeatist is inclined to depend on the conservative potential of his fundamental wager concerning social and political tendencies.

If the preceding analysis holds, and Kissinger did not continue the effort to structurally reform the international system by rearranging existing forces for the purpose of releasing new forces in support of the essentially conservative objectives of U.S. foreign policy, to be pursued through leadership in global equilibrium, then his conservative statecraft was not Bismarckian in basic philosophy any more than it was in grand strategy. A philosophic posture of defiance did not inspire a creative handling of the mechanical and organic dimensions of international politics. Instead, a form of Spenglerian despair in Kissinger's philosophy of history (regarding the "West") commingled with the special kind of perverse Metternichian optimism in political philosophy to rationalize an approach that was essentially defeatist and bade fair to be ultimately self-defeating. In order to make sense, the approach had to be predicated on the sufficiency of U.S.-Soviet détente for repose and on its utility as a sanctuary for combating radical change by means including occasional "repressions" (thus, with all due differences, Chile was for Kissinger what Naples had been for Metternich). If pessimism about the West compelled détente, the implied optimism about the "East" (comprising the Communist great powers and the Third World) permitted it. The danger was that the implicit wager would not work: that the dislocative consequences of the détente strategy in the West would further aggravate the conditions that had prompted the original pessimism about it, while these same dislocations—along with drift in regard to the Third World—would eliminate the bases for the relative optimism concerning the "East." That is to say, strategic shortcomings in relation to both of the geopolitical realms would feed into the philosophic duality, fulfilling the pessimistic strand and frustrating the potential behind the optimistic one.

In such circumstances, an excessive (and growing?) dependence on détente with the Soviet Union in great-power relations, combined with strategic passivity in the Third World only sporadically relieved by efforts to pacify conventional turmoils and repress "revolutionary" ones, could degenerate into a growing dependence on Soviet abidance by détente. In conditions in which the détente policy itself weakened the bases for its gradual development into a combination of local *ad hoc* ententes and system-wide devolution, the pressures would grow for the carrier of Spenglerian despair to abandon the Metternichian quest for stability and find a more effective expression in the Kaunitzian strategy for conflict. Trying to shift from accommodation with the Soviet Union to a sweepingly devolutionary alliance with China, and any other still available countervailing force, would then mean attempting a major diplomatic revolution as the last-resort remedy for debilitating détente and its illegitimate offspring, competitive *détentisme*.

II

Even if it were to be agreed that the United States is or ought to be engaged in a gradual strategic retreat from empire to equilibrium, the question still would be whether its role is to be leadership in multistate equilibrium politics or dependence on continuing equilibrium within a two-power diplomatic system—the first anticipating somewhat upon the lagging "hard" aspects of the international system and the second lagging behind its "softer" aspects. The two possibilities imply two different structures of the international system and two different views of the evolutionary stage of the United States as a power: a power in either case "declining" from the previously dominant position but one endowed under the two scenarios with different degrees of resilience and residual strength for determining the nature of the new position and the new setting relative to the previous ones. In both historical and analytic or structural terms, the basic choice is between the diplomatic systems of Bismarck and Metternich (with the Kaunitzian reversal as the threatening presence mainly in the latter's background). A clue to the right choice is to be found in an indigenous American precedent for the transition from empire to equilibrium; the correct choice follows more significantly from the weighing of determinants implicit in the contemporary state of the international system on the one hand and in America's developmental stage on the other. The key background questions are: is the U.S. foreign policy consigned to Kissinger's quasi-Metternichian or neo-Metternichian system for good, because it is too late to apply the Bismarckian one (given America's moral-material decadence), or is it so consigned only for some more time, because it is too early for the Bismarckian system (given the structural deficiencies in the international system)?

What are, once again, the basic features of the three diplomatic systems which crystallize differently the two fundamental ways of conservative philosophy and statecraft in behalf of powers in need of different mechanical responses to different organic predicaments? If, as was pointed out, the Kaunitzian system of radical realignment stands between the Metternichian and Bismarckian on the mechanical-organic dimension (as one suited for the relatively declining but still strong and militant power), it is closer to the Bismarckian system on the defiance-defeatism spectrum of conservative philosophy when it is adopted from still-substantial strength (as it was, only in the international segment, for the internally secure prerevolutionary mid-eighteenth-century original). The Kaunitzian *système* moves toward and even beyond the Metternichian one on the scale of conservative despondency, however, when it represents only the compulsive, aggressively self-defensive spasm of resistance to the unavoidable consummation by a power in the later or last stages of decline.[1]

Transposed to the present, the Bismarckian system means counterpoising the Communist powers (and any additional greater powers) for two basic purposes. On the primary global plane, the purpose is to promote and then stabilize a multipower international system rather than any particular situation (such as the U.S.-Soviet détente). The specific positive objective is to perpetuate U.S. leadership in the new equilibrium system, preclude a permanent recoalescence of China and the Soviet Union, and promote the rise of Western Europe (or, alternatively, West Germany) and eventually Japan to at least a supporting or secondary independent role in great-power diplomacy. A neo-Bismarckian multipower system generates its objectives by giving China a stake in independence and stimulating Western Europe (and Japan) to seek independence; the first impedes reintegration of the Sino-Soviet "bloc" in a more equal alliance, and the second fosters a deintegration of the American "bloc" into an association more contingent as well as equal. The regional plane is a derivative of the global great-power plane in the Bismarckian worldview, as great powers maneuver for and around interdependent strategies for composing explosive regional conflicts on the basis of political settlements with either hegemonial or equilibrium overtones while condoning —and even promoting—regional balance-of-power systems on the basis of hierarchical stratification.

If, ideally, the Bismarckian system generates its positive structural objectives, as it were, spontaneously, the neo-Metternichian system, in the gloomiest view, engenders its inherently negative possible consequences with near-equal automaticity. This happens if progressing normalization with all Communist powers (including the Soviet Union, China, and some lesser powers) proves incompatible with specialized détente-accommodation with the Soviet Union; or if even the subtlest orchestration of policy emphases along the differential normalization-détente-entente spectrum proves insufficient either to offset the potential of the two-power accommodation to dislocate or debilitate the power base of the

---

[1] On foreign-policy "stages" see Liska, *War and Order* (Baltimore: Johns Hopkins University Press, 1968), pp. 4–11.

more conservative of the two principal parties or, again, to contain the consequences of regionally originated disruptions for the two-power accommodation itself. Détente policy will suffer in exact proportion to its inaptness to deal with continuing differences on specific issues of geopolitical import at least as effectively as it can deal with the broad issues—be they abstract, symbolic, or long-term developmental—clustering around primacy and parity, repose and revolution. In that respect, the Middle Eastern apple of discord between the United States and the Soviet Union in the current neo-Metternichian setting has been the equivalent of the Balkans (or the "Near East") between Russia and Austria in the Metternichian and, increasingly, immediately post-Metternichian context. If, however, conservative appeasement between great powers founders on the reefs of either local antagonisms or deepening derangements for one power only, the logical response is recoil from conciliation to the Kaunitzian prescription for reconquest of the lost asset or redressal of an eroding relative position.

Although the lost asset was territorial in Kaunitz's case (Silesia), it need not be necessarily so. Metternich regressed from France to Great Britain and on to Russia as the principal conservative ally for Austria, and the regression progressively decreased Austria's potential or actual independence and status as a great power. The United States has had a nearly equivalent range of possible principal allies. A restored Western Europe *sans* de Gaulle (equaling Bonapartist France *sans* Napoleon for Metternich) was the proper ally for a dominant position vis-à-vis both of the Communist great powers: China (equaling Great Britain) for the militant containment of Russia and Soviet Russia (equaling Tsarist Russia) for conservative repose. A successor of Metternich's felt subsequently compelled to switch back to France and Britain against Russia, in an effort to recoup the loss in position by means of a modified replica of the Kaunitzian original. Similarly, Kissinger's successors may have to revert to the power or powers neglected in the contemporary neo-Metternichian system while liquidating a design that had not fulfilled its essential purpose or had worked in favor of one party (as both the Austro-British and the Franco-Prussian alliances had done in one way or another). The degree of the damage previously done would determine whether the reversion would be only part of the way and peaceful, thus restoring a flexible Bismarckian system as it had been adumbrated in the early Nixon-Kissinger strategy, or else would be integral and militant, thus realizing to the full the perverse Kaunitzian potential of the Metternichian design. The doctrinal basis for such reversion (to Bismarck) or reversal (*à la* Kaunitz) has been provided by Kissinger himself in his stated opposition to having any great power (i.e., the Soviet Union) exploit détente for the pursuit of predominance regionally or, by extension, globally.

If the evolution in American foreign policy is from Metternich to Bismarck, i.e., to controlled revision of two-power détente in favor of more widely extended devolution, American foreign policy will reenact an American precedent for the retreat from empire to equilibrium. The home-grown antecedent for such a posture is the "large policy" of active great-power diplomacy with which Theodore Roosevelt followed up his prepresidential activity as a chief exponent of overseas empire. The sequence, writ large, has since been reproduced in the post–World War II evolution of U.S. foreign policy (and of both Nixon and Kissinger themselves). The Rooseveltian great-power policy sought status and influence without the costs of any further territorial acquisitions or politico-military interventions. It did so with the aid of diplomatic activism symbolically sustained by occasional naval displays and including mediation for peace (most conspicuously between Russia and Japan). The dominant bias was against an irreversible preemption of the American title to global primacy by either Russia or Japan in the Asian Pacific sphere and by Germany or Britain in the Atlantic sphere in particular. If the resulting special biases shifted as between the first two, however, they soon settled into a fixed anti-German and thus pro-British mold with respect to the second pair.

The consummation of the Rooseveltian vision of American world power in a setting of multipower *Weltpolitik* was postponed to the second try in the present by intervening deviations. The departures included Taftian nonstrategic economism (the "dollar diplomacy"), Wilsonian institutionalism (the League of Nations) opposed by Lodgean unilateralism, and Harding-to-Hoover's (and early FDR's) isolationism. In the guise of their neo-variants, these attitudes have resurfaced in the contemporary environment of American foreign policy whenever proponents of a revitalized economism impugned Kissinger's restrictively noneconomic diplomacy while Atlantic institutionalists deplored his unilateralism as part of a quarrel of schools over the best means for containing any new spell of American isolationism. In contrast to the present situation, however, the costfree Rooseveltian great-powerism was buoyed up by a beneficient combination of attributes since departed. They singled out the United States as both marginal to the diplomatic arena of the day and prospectively salient as the rising world power. The first attribute bestowed upon the United States a leeway superior to that of any other power, while the second one made it the object of equally assiduous wooing by all the powers without lasting exception. In so abnormal a situation, any deficiency in will and capacity for effective intervention was more than made up for by the arrogant self-confidence of the self-designated heirs of all the ages.

A bit more effort—in the expenditure of both intellectual and moral energy and material resource—has since become necessary to protect the essential parts of the American inheritance internationally. An earlier political generation could express itself through such acts as the Hay Notes, mere paper reservations of positions to be effectively occupied in a later phase as part of a pro-American devolution of empire. That privilege has since been replaced by pressures to erect defenses, some of them only paper-thin, against uncontrolled and adverse devolution of power (less responsibility?) from the American to the next empire or empires—global or local, military or economic. The collective American psyche has been suspended between the internally generated craving for constriction and the externally fomented pressures for reassertion or even reexpansion. The domestic dilemma reflected a radical mis-fit between the (low) morale and the (still major) material assets intrinsic to the American polity. American policy abroad, in turn, has wavered on the path of transition from empire to equilibrium leadership for reasons having to do with both basic concept and routine implementation of the dominant conservative design. The international system has been simultaneously shaken by the latest installments of the Middle Eastern conflict and the (apparently) last one of the Southeast Asian conflict; and it has been strained by the successive waves of diffusion and lopsided reconcentration of economic power, while international economics and ecology moved into operative purview of high policy filling the partial vacuum of conflict and concept in the political arena. But the issue of the "fit" of Kissinger's diplomatic system involved nonetheless first and foremost the traditionally familiar aspects of power balances and conflict configurations among the major states: disparities in the evolutionary stages of individual powers and in the equilibrium structures of the different regions were still more critical than any supposedly new spirit of foreign policy and nature of the international system.

If America's stage of material and moral development is used as the main criterion for determining the fit-ness of the dominant diplomatic strategy, the case for a Metternichian approach must rest on the belief that the United States is no longer capable of sustaining the more demanding Bismarckian one. Accordingly, quite apart from the question of whether the Bismarckian system was or was not "obsolete" in terms of the contemporary nature of international politics and foreign policy, it could be deemed to be anachronistic for a power in an advanced stage of relative and absolute decline. Since the United States of today could not be easily equated with the Austria of Metternich's day, the contention that it could not reenact with greater effect the Bismarck-like strategies of Theodore Roosevelt might rest more accurately on identifying contemporary America with Great Britain in the period roughly coincident with the first Roosevelt's official tenure. Discounting differences, the United States would then equal turn-of-the-century Britain as an overextended and declining imperial power, beset by the rise of rival powers in the central balance of power and facing, in addition to a deteriorating economic situation, the problem of proliferation in the "ultimate" weapon of the age (nuclear versus naval), acceleration of disruptive tendencies in peripheral regions (the Third World in general versus Egypt and South Africa), and increasingly centrifugal tendencies among the principal associates (America's major allies versus Britain's white dominions). In such a situation, the embarrassed power will legitimately look to easing its burdens while hoping to preserve the vital assets. The British formula was to combine accommodation with the principal challenger for succession and wider devolution of responsibilities and capacities onto other major powers. The all-important question concerned then, as it does now, the choice of the principal partner in accommodation and the assortment and synchronization of the accommodational with the devolutionary strategy.

With respect to accommodation, Britain vacillated between Germany and the United States and opted for the American aspirant to imperial succession as one with whom to compose first and principally. In the analogy between one-time Britain and the contemporary United States, the related question is whether the détente policy with the Soviet Union is to be compared with the finally futile groping for an Anglo-German entente or with the accomplished Anglo-American understanding. To be properly illuminated, the analogical issue has to be approached from the vantage point of structure, policy, and function. Structurally, the Soviet Union can be readily equated with Imperial Germany as the dominant land or continental power in Europe with developing naval ambitions that are challenging to the previously dominant sea or maritime power. The more the contemporary Soviet Union goes naval, however, without American opposition in conditions when the land-sea power cleavage is structurally less important than it used to be,[2] the more does Soviet Russia resemble the United States of 1900 rather than the Germany of that same period. The structural similarities are then of a more specific kind. They find expression less in an arms race and more in geopolitically conditioned competition in policy over the balance of access to the fragmented geographic underbelly of the rising power. The underbelly was the Central American-cum-Carribean complex in the Anglo-American setting as compared with the Middle Eastern-cum-Persian Gulf complex in the American-Soviet one. The related pretension of the ascendant power was (and presumably is) to curtail the previously dominant world power's access to the relevant continental land mass—Britain's to the western hemisphere and America's to Eur-Asia respectively—and, ultimately perhaps, to secure its control. The structural parallel is confirmed by policy, insofar as both accommodations (the Anglo-American and the American-Soviet) unfolded in function of the very contest itself over the respective land bridge (Central America and the Middle East), over the critical passageway (the Isthmian canal

[2] See p. 18.

and the Suez canal), and over the adjacent waters (Atlantic-Pacific and Mediterranean-Indian Ocean, respectively). The United States has accommodated with the Soviet Union while accepting almost as fully as Britain had done with respect to the then United States the necessity to avoid an "ultimate" conflict or confrontation over stabilizing a parity agreement on the substantively important and symbolically overarching "underbelly" issue. But, whereas a parity arrangement was only provisionally acceptable to the ascendant U.S. in the earlier context, it has—perhaps only provisionally—not yet been accepted by American policy in the present one.

Conversely, still in policy terms, just as Great Britain recoiled from composing with Germany on the specific issue of a common approach to China and East Asia generally, so the United States has been soft-pedaling the normalization with China and has arrested it well short of its becoming a factor in the approach to the contemporary problem of Germany and East Europe—as well as of Southeast Asia. Only a deepening Sino-American accord was, however, capable of containing the Soviet Union, just as only a serious Anglo-German accommodation would have contained the United States in both hemispheres. In actuality, the American distaste for an Anglo-German accommodation was a factor in Britain's deciding against Germany. Similarly, the degree of effective intimacy in U.S.-Chinese relations that was consistent with the Soviet conception of détente could not but be a factor regulating Sino-American normalization as long as U.S.-Soviet détente was assigned absolute priority.

The Anglo-American accommodation proved to be an illusion from the British viewpoint, since it did not initiate the transition to an Anglo-American global condominium. But it fulfilled the most daring American expectations of imperial succession. This raises —following the structural and policy considerations—the functional issue: Accommodation for what? If accommodation with the principal challenger is a policy of retreat from empire, its result may be transfer of primacy to the aspirant. Any danger or appearance of this happening via the U.S.-Soviet détente confirms the analogy with Anglo-American accommodation. If détente policy is, on the other hand, part of an effort at retention of essential empire with only minimal American retrenchment, then the more apt analogy is with the Anglo-German *attempts* at accommodation. By such devices as the Moscow Declaration pledging joint promotion of regional peace, the United States would be asking the Soviet Union to do world-wide what Germany refused to do for Britain in Asia: pull (British) chestnuts out of the fire without any concurrent redistribution of geopolitically significant assets. Just as accommodation is liable to collapse over American resistance if détente is the road to decadence, détente as the way to cost-free American dominion would be doomed from the Soviet viewpoint. The remaining third possibility is accommodation which, while implementing retreat from empire, avoids transfer of imperial primacy for transformation of the international system. This alternative ought, in principle, to be acceptable to both parties. It raises, however, most directly the practical issue of how to assort the accommodation and the devolution strategies. The issue points to some further analogies between one-time Britain and today's United States and also to some major differences.

In the British case, accommodation with the United States was combined with devolutionary strategy by way of Britain's new alliance with Japan and, in subsequent chain reaction, ententes with France and Russia. Along with these efforts to relieve demands on British seapower were the not-so-successful efforts to share and coordinate imperial security obligations with the self-governing white dominions. The American equivalent would be devolution in favor of tightened ties with China and loosened ties with Western Europe and Japan. The devolutionary reinsurance did not work for Britain with respect to the United States because it was bent almost entirely into service against Germany. It worked for the then United States for the same reasons. The Anglo-American accommodation had a specific extraneous focus or target in German ambitions, which, while being of more immediate import for the British, were opposed with comparatively greater ideological fervor by leading Americans. The U.S.-Soviet détente has had no comparable one-power focus. The two powers have shared, if anything, only a very diffuse extraneous focus in global stability and internal economies, differently interpreted and pursued by each. Joint preoccupation with a third power meant that Britain could not effectively control the balance of costs and benefits of her accommodation with the United States through the devolutionary strategy. Instead, the devolutionary strategy, involving alignment with France and Russia, promoted polarization in the central balance of power which made Britain in due course wholly dependent on the United States.

By contrast, the absence of a common great-power enemy in the U.S.-Soviet détente, and the fact that China has been at odds more with the Soviet Union than with the United States, has strengthened the American position in the détente relationship over against what was Britain's. This systemic advantage reinforces the favorable difference in relative inherent strengths between a contemporary United States, with or without principal allies, and one-time Great Britain, with or without feasible empire coordination. The United States has been, therefore, in principle able to regulate the cost-benefit implications of the U.S.-Soviet accommodation as long as it kept active and further developed the devolutionary complement: i.e., as long as China in particular was both available because it was strong and independent enough, and was not antagonistic and aggressive because it was too strong or no longer fully independent in policy. That is to say, the *immediate* danger for the United States from the détente-accommodation policy has not been polarization in the central balance of conventional power comprising the three great powers. It consists, instead, in an erosion of that balance if China's involvement were to wane and Western Europe's or Japan's failed to wax, and in polarization of a parallel balance along South-North lines comprising "revolutionary" power under China's leadership. Only in the longer term would the conventional balance of power be in danger of re-polarization from an irresistibly ascendant Soviet Russia, if she constrained China into an offensive alliance or if a countervailing defensive Sino-American alliance was still available as an active option.

III

The only remedy to any one form of derangement between the détente strategy and a devolutionary strategy is to continue developing the Bismarckian system of multi-power counterpoising. It is the necessary corrective to the trends toward, or the dangers of, the Metternichian system of *de facto* dependence on one power.

To do so is not beyond the material capacity of the contemporary United States measured by the yardstick of the distribution of power and conflicts relative to the two Communist great powers. It is even less infeasible in the light of the comparison with one-time Britain in *her* systemic context. A reactivation of the Bismarckian strand would thus not be anachronistic in the sense of coming "too late" in terms of American capabilities. Is it, by contrast, premature? Is the international system not ready for it because the two Communist powers have not yet evolved sufficiently conventional stakes and strategies? Or is the configuration of power and conflict not yet sufficiently crystallized or diversified, partially as a result of the just-mentioned impediment? The existence of a gap or mis-fit between a full-blown Bismarckian diplomatic system and the contemporary international system was too explicitly asserted previously to be now denied.[3] It has also been established, however, that the rightness of a diplomatic system is not wholly a matter of immediate payoff but is also a matter of vindication in the long run. And it has been argued that creative statecraft effectively attempts to narrow any such gap or attenuate any mis-fit. If the key purpose is orderly transition from empire to leadership in equilibrium, moreover, any degree to which a full-fledged equilibrium strategy is validly thought to be premature in terms of both actual risks or possible results implies the same degree to which the relinquishment of imperial resources would be likewise premature—and counterproductive. The principal imperial resource is the capacity for militarily backed—or implemented—intervention. This means one thing for narrowing any gap on the great-power or global level of a devolution-for-détente diplomacy and another for the lesser-power or regional level.

Among the great powers, the residual imperial resource is necessary for sustaining confrontational or coercive diplomacy as the indispensable complement of both concessionary and concert-type diplomacy. In general and on the regional issues in the Middle East and Southeast Asia in particular, the main object of such diplomacy has been to secure "fair" Soviet cooperation in *ad hoc* concert for a "fair" return (toward parity), while securing China against the Soviet Union as a condition of her self-assertion in

[3] See pp. 45ff.

Southeast Asia (and Eastern Europe) against the Soviet Union regionally and for multi-power equilibrium diplomacy globally. On the lesser-state level, the immediate purpose of the well-assorted concessionary-and-coercive diplomacy for equilibrium is to enable the United States to contain abuses of both political and economic power. The purpose of containing the sources of excessive regional or global disorders consequent on unchecked abuses is not only immediate self-protection. It is also the creation of both the basic disposition and the basic precondition for releasing genuinely dynamic local forces into evolving increasingly autonomous regional balance-of-power orders.

An appropriate diplomacy with great powers and smaller states might stimulate the major Western European allies (and, in due course, the Japanese ally) by exposing them to the risks and opportunities of an active three-power configuration globally and involving them in the regional devolutionary process. Such involvement would be attractive if an active association with a manifest U.S. capacity for intervention against flagrant abuses of power engendered material rewards and immaterial (status and morale) payoffs and substituted these for the material and status costs of the alternative: unwarranted identification with previously uncoordinated U.S. actions. The costs of the alternative have included the partial and potentially divisive European reactions and remedies for the consequences of being so identified; and the identification itself took place in part at least because the economically strong minor powers needed a hostage for American good behavior in the more vulnerable Western European (and Japanese) economies even more than the Soviet Union has continued to need the Western European hostage in the nuclear-strategic arena. There may prove to be no other escape for Western Europe from all of the three threatening hegemonies (American, Soviet, "Arab") than by the door of an improved self-defense capacity also as the basis for a more "equal" Atlantic confederacy capable of primarily sea- and air-borne action in the Mediterranean and related seas and littorals. Such confederacy would not aim to realize at this late date and in a new guise the expectations of shared supremacy that the British had once attached to their accommodation with the United States. But it could be sufficiently well-coordinated to permit joint military action of a limited-conventional kind outside

Europe and sufficiently loose and flexible to permit parallel or independent diplomatic action of a strategic kind. Whereas the joint military effort would blunt the hegemonic implications for Western Europe of a U.S. military intervention in behalf of primarily European economic interests in the Third World, a more solidly based European capacity for independent diplomatic action would, among other things, weaken somewhat the collusive implications of the U.S.-Soviet accommodation for China's politico-military interests in Asia.

It may not be too far-fetched to assume that, continuing to take the "oil crisis" as an example, a conspicuous U.S.-European military planning activity might in itself suffice to offset the immediate disparities in economic leverage, without seriously impeding the prospects from alternative approaches to the crisis once the initial hostile reaction had been absorbed. In the extreme case of direct action, a more-than-token European participation would be required to remove the prime foundation for European objections to a forcible American intervention: i.e., the objection that such action would reaffirm the American hold on Western Europe in both the short and the long run. Whether implemented in contingency planning or in crisis action, the renewal of comradeship in arms for a practical and practicable purpose would invest the joint activity with the potential for vitalizing—by one stroke, as it were—both European politico-military identity and the overarching spirit of Atlantic solidarity in the last resort. There are not many ways to pursue the two disparate objectives simultaneously and undo the lingering consequences of Suez 1956. Moreover, a visible posture of determination to defend oneself under economic siege would reassure China about the continued viability of the West in general —and Western Europe in particular—as a counterpoise to Soviet Russia. The desert wind would cease buffeting at will the Western city; there would be some teeth again to the tiger. Japan would know more surely than before where to look in the short run (and to what means, in the long) for the security of her vital supplies. A new period of diplomatic creativity might even ensue from the combined politico-economic and politico-military Middle Eastern crisis, as it did earlier from the Vietnam war, amplifying thus any relief gained in the economic sector. In such conditions, "power" in its different elements would have been moderately diffused and the lines of conflicts diversified further away from the East-West axis, even while the South-North confrontation was put on the agenda in earnest as something to be attended to by both classic and newly constructive means before Southern miscalculations, nourished by the pliancy of the industrial world, will have forced the West to shed all restraint on the full use of its latent strengths.

No single military measure, any more than any particular diplomatic maneuver, can reshape the international system and impress upon it a determinate constellation. But any reassertion of the American imperial strain outside Western Europe and Japan would place the United States in a better position for the long-term balancing of power against power. It would move the United States closer to the Bismarckian system of equilibrium leadership and spare it the Metternichian pursuit of universal concert from a position of timorous weakness, while enlarging its range of choices in the Kaunitzian perspective of intensified conflict. Whichever way the events may move, the future will be circumscribed by the extremes of multi-power equipoise and one-power hegemony and, within that range, by the three prototypical diplomatic systems. Together, structures of power and diplomatic strategies of the major states will, in the last resort, determine the course and control the consequences of only partially novel "transnational" inter-dependence and inter-nation "equality." Only when the relation between old and new determinants has been reversed actually in periods of serious conflict or concert rather than fictitiously in the doldrums of the secular cycle's détente phase will the Bismarckian statesman have cause to sign off into the annals of antiquarian history.

On the other hand, as long as the tripolar international system and the triangular strategies remain what they have been recently, the mere shadow of a Bismarckian diplomatic system will survive on the parallel weaknesses of the major powers even more than on their counterpoised strengths. It will do so within an international system in which diffusion of power and conflicts has not been systematically promoted any more than the limited margins for compensation have been exploited by a statecraft contingent for success upon, and superficially dedicated to, both. It is no comfort to note the possibility that the internal limitations of Kissinger's statecraft only compounded the domestically imposed limits on material means under which it labored. And it is an unreliable comfort to note that the weaknesses of the major states, if parallel, are not identical in kind and tend to complement one another for transient appeasement while provisionally neutralizing the gusto of each for massive self-assertion; and that power, conflicts, and compensations have acquired new—if apparently ever-changing—dimensions which for a time can replace functionally and blunt politically whatever deficiencies may exist in their more traditional varieties. The comfort is unreliable because, in such circumstances, any present stability of the international system is, and will remain, at the mercy of the first inordinate assertion of power by any one of the major states—or, indeed, of any group of fleetingly favored minor ones. As for the United States itself, having presumably ceased to be unquestionably hegemonial or imperial, it is not yet weak enough to be Metternichian and not desperate enough to fight off a grasping challenger to have to be integrally Kaunitzian. Nor, since it is no longer either the bright promise or the spoiled infant of international politics, can it be effortlessly and profitably (Theodore) Rooseveltian.

If it is clear what the United States of today is not, however, it is far from equally certain what it is and is to become. The basic challenge posed for both the Nixon-Kissinger team and its successors was one of retreating from a momentarily untenable foreign-policy position into a posture that would sustain vital stakes at less cost. There was more than one path to this widely accepted objective; and the crossroads were demarcated with both tactical and conceptual choices. Their deliberate or unwitting resolution would cumulatively determine the direction taken, without insuring that it would lead to the proposed destination.

If the object is retreat or retrenchment from a dominant or paramount position, the key question is less "how much?" than "where to?" The reallocation of to-be-reduced material resources is, in the process, subject to risks over different time-spans. The desired destination may well be, we have noted, leadership in successor equilibrium as an alternative to another's imperial succession. The strategic pathway will be beset by risks and consequent responsibilities for the risk-taker that are either immediate for the strategist or can be delayed to his successors; risks and responsibilities that can be assumed near-instantly in shaping conditions or delayed to a supposedly later maturity of supporting conditions. The basic choice is then between deferred gradualism and grandiose diplomacy. The first involves sacrificing control over the end result for control over the next step. It can assume the form of defusing a military situation locally, as a preliminary to gradually evolved pacific political settlement; or it can aim globally at lowering the level of the strategic-military deterrent balance with the major-power adversary, as one of the preliminaries to an eventual progressive devolution within a wider scope. In such an approach, "dramatic" solutions are rejected for a more stately "choreography."[4] The danger is that procedural delays will end in defeat for the strategy's material objective, and that deferred gradualism will precipitate immobilism. By contrast, the practitioner of the more daring or grandiose strategy accepts the risks of the strategy's misfiring almost instantly in order to accelerate the process. He sacrifices control over the next step in order to foreshorten the time frame sufficiently to maximize control over the forces ultimately determining the desired transformation. Volatility in the short run is the price paid for the greater chance of substituting consolidation for immobility in the long. In moral terms, the fact that the grandiose statesman cannot help assuming responsibility for the outcome effaces any taint of reckless irresponsibility that might inhere in the procedure; whereas in the gradualist's case, prudence in manner will nearly guarantee diluted responsibility for the final shape of the matter wrought by policy.

The difference between immobility and consolidation suggests two kinds of stability, which correspond to the difference between repose and resilience. It is possible to stabilize an international system in depth by consolidating a flexible equilibrium system as the increasingly routinized dominant procedure; or a given power distribution can be stabilized superficially by the transient suspension of conflict. The first entails an even diffusion of the stake that unequally powerful and unevenly evolving states acquire in the dynamic equilibrium system; the second would perpetuate or only marginally adjust the stake that the favored major states have in even an unbalanced configuration of power. The first system aims

---

[4] Kissinger's words. See his "The Viet Nam Negotiations," *Foreign Affairs*, January 1969, pp. 217, 218.

at self-correcting resilience, and the second aims at repose to correct through restraint the consequences of prior exertion or to weaken present impediments to future exertion. The quest for political repose without supporting resilience risks unleashing pressures for an abrupt reversal of diplomatic strategy or alignment from weakness, however. By the same token, material retrenchment in similar conditions risks engendering strains and dislocations that will release pressures for remedial reexpansion. A stabilized multi-power equilibrium system, as part of post-imperial American interactions with increasingly postrevolutionary Communist (and other) powers, has become the surest safeguard against reversal of one-sided détente and against reexpansion into one-power imperium regionally or globally, even while the manifest capacity for such reexpansion may in some circumstances be the surest warranty of progress toward the desired kind of equilibrium.

If détente is desirable only if combined with wider devolution which reinsures it on both the great- and middle-power levels, the question still is, "What kind of détente and devolution?" Détente as a matter of appeasement pursued by the previously dominant or possessing power or powers occurs, almost by definition, from a relatively superior prior position: what is less certain is that it occurs also from continuing inherent and situational strength. This raises several questions. On whose terms does détente take place generally, as contrasted with the specific terms reflecting tangible or identifiable comparative costs and benefits? Within what sustaining systemic environment does détente take place: one that structurally redresses the psychological disadvantage for the relatively receding power while reinsuring it against a rate of demands for change that would be productive of the détente's failure, or one that does not? The issue of the end goal applies to appeasement as it does to retrenchment, but more concretely: if the object is equilibrium, then is it the equilibrium of a "dual alliance" inverting militant bipolarity into the outlines of an (inversely unbalanced?) conservative partnership if not condominium, or is it a multi-power equilibrium evolved by concessionary-coercive diplomacy intent upon dissolving the stalemating effect of residual military bipolarity? And if the goal is not a staid condominium, is détente to grow into entente by gradual system-wide progression involving two powers ever more in a generalized (functional) cooperation and in ever less (political) competition with one another; or, as earlier discussion suggested, is entente to aggregate mechanically, as it were, by way of concerts on specific (and geopolitically critical) issues with different powers and with the aid of *ad hoc* confrontational or coercive diplomacy? Is entente to be, again, deferred and gradual or, in its several parts, immediate and grandiose?

If accommodation from a superior position entails concessions, are they to be—or can they be—uncompensated?; and if détente from strength entails a wider devolution, can the latter be wholly uncontrolled? It is likely that both requirements, compensation and control, can be met best by synchronizing the détente and devolution processes across the international system—i.e., by not having devolution follow détente selectively sector by sector. A system-wide approach to détente and devolution would thus differ from the sectorial approach to détente and entente while complementing it operationally. Concessions will automatically mean loss of assets, and devolution, loss of direct control, if they occur separately and in isolation. Just as isolation of specific problems leads to a diplomacy that shuttles restlessly from one crisis to another, isolating approaches to the general problem of retrenchment and reequilibration from one another will tend to paralyze effort by creating the impression of cumulating costs. If deferral of devolution is "bad" because it confines two-power détente within the relentless boundaries of the zero-sum game, the dispersal of devolution simultaneously with détente can be "good" if the wider restructuring transfers the two-power accommodation into a larger framework of concessionary cost-benefit calculations.

Hence the argument that détente with the Soviet Union is safer if there is concurrent devolution in favor of China and Western Europe (and Japan). And devolution in Europe and Asia can be thus made safer without becoming uncontrollable: safer, because it consolidates the distracting pressure on the Soviet Union from the East in the form of an internationally fully integrated China; and residually controllable, because a systemically reinsured U.S.-Soviet détente creates a policy leeway for the United States that can be bargained, with Chinese encouragement, into control over the outermost boundaries of the enhanced Western European and Japanese autonomy. The basic principle applies also to the next-lower level of the hierarchically stratified plural balance-of-power system. A system-wide devolutionary setting is safer and more controllable as regards the behavior of the regional middle powers than are isolated instances of devolution individually. Inasmuch as the middle powers are a unified class in terms of status, commitment to devolution across the board tends to slacken their hostile defensive reaction vis-à-vis the great powers, which is rooted in resentment at being artificially equalized with the truly small states. Moreover, inasmuch as the middle powers are also and more significantly a diversified aggregation of separate and often competing entities, they will individually require different forms of great-power backing against one another in intra- and inter-regional equilibrium systems and against different and changing great powers. The consequent dynamic has the potential for being ultimately stabilizing for the international system as a whole. It would be propitious to a United States acting as the leader in global equilibrium least likely to seek direct control in any one particular region. And it would tend to secure even for a less favorably situated United States some middle-power friends, as they recoiled from other associations or antagonisms and compensated thereby for the loss of middle powers defecting from the United States in temporary response to past experiences. Like the counterpoising of several great powers, a devolutionary process in several places at once reduces both the requisite efforts at control and the material and other costs of containment or control to the net margin of hostile power or incompatible intentions emerging from the largely self-neutralizing dynamic.

By contrast, the devolutionary strategy augments demands on the social resources of political intelligence expended in monitoring and, if need be, manipulating the process. There is thus, unavoidably, a tradeoff between different kinds of costs, not least in a strategy aiming at the reduction of the most burdensome material costs. The cost alternatives have been illustrated in connection with the discussion of different approaches to peacemaking in Southeast Asia.[5] There, too, was the most immediate occasion for assessing the ideal cost of ceasing to implement past commitments. Such costs must be measured against the cost of having the indefi-

[5] See p. 56.

116

nitely continuing formal observance of past commitments unpro-
ductively impede new configurations and relationships—both of
which may well have been rendered possible by previously honor-
ing the commitments and made necessary by implementing them
with only limited efficacy. In other words, the system-wide costs of
breaking promises to allied élites must be weighed against the costs
of blocking positive performance over time; moral responsibility
must in the end be tempered with concern for political results—
even while it can be discounted for the reasonable assumption that
the local élites themselves have acted out of self-interest at all
times and are obligated to adjust goals to the capacity for self-
dependence at some point in time. A diminished confidence in
American commitments that had been incurred in the "imperial"
setting might well promote erosion of restraints on forms of behavior antagonistic to that setting. That setting has been renounced,
however, in principle, as no longer serviceable in its entirety. This
stripped of any compensatory advantage, and consequently magni-
fied the costs of, the policy of automatically upholding prior
understandings if they constrain effective American efforts to adjust and adapt to the emergent post-imperial setting. The fact that
the issue comprises genuine dilemmas eliminates any one simple
response—including one in favor of American promises and credibility—unless, indeed, a rigid moral stance in the present were to
degenerate into a political device for passing onto the future the
consequences of the failure to deflect past policies from their abandoned original goals while there is still time.

The tradeoff between costs means that material costs are *in the
final analysis* reducible only in exchange for another kind of cost
and liability. It is of course possible to reduce material costs directly. Armaments costs can be lowered by a combination of co-
operative arms-limitation agreements with the Soviet Union and
interallied competition over arms sale agreements with lesser powers. The entire détente policy can be calculated to reduce material
costs of containment by buying off the Soviet Union: reduce pressure by reducing competition with the aid of commercial deals and
agreements one-sidedly favorable to the Soviets. If the specific
costs and benefits of détente are not evenly balanced, however, this
kind of direct cost reduction is liable to involve American losses in
either relative material standing, formal status, or both. The very

importance of cost-equalization between only two and differently unequal powers, and the near-insurmountable difficulty of a reliable determination of what constitutes equality, will serve to undermine the détente policy in the longer run. Hence the importance of saving on material costs not so much by onesided transfers or by reduction of two-power competition as by expanding the range of parties to conflict and concert within a many-sided systemic transformation. In an expanded constellation there is more scope for concessions to be diversified and either reciprocally neutralized or otherwise compensated. Material costs in upholding essential positions are reduced when one-power management or an unmanageable reciprocal outbidding by two powers in the military arms- or economic growth-races, or in the race for third-party favors, are transformed into the manipulation of net margins. The overall costs are thus not reduced, but the balance of material and immaterial costs is changed.

The fundamental tradeoff in the expanded and diversified setting is between resource and risk. As the demand on resource declines in a flexible equilibrium situation, and with it the cost in more or less well-managed material assets, the risk implicit in more or less well-conceived strategic or tactical movement grows in proportion. A reduction in costs involving material resource may be imposed —as it was in the United States—by domestic constraints, in part due to economic and social disruptions; it is then up to the conservative international statesman to assume the additional compensating risks in such a way as to minimize the deranging impact of the domestic instabilities on foreign policy. It is, in principle, not possible to preserve essential interests and positions while saving on both resources and risks. A statecraft or statesman seeking to create the contrary impression is merely deferring the moment of accounting while eschewing the immediate responsibility for facing up to the dilemma and implementing its practical implications. In fact, if he sidesteps the resource-risk tradeoff, he merely shifts to a different and supreme kind of tradeoff: between the gamble on an audacious transforming strategy and the wager on the conformity of a prudential conservative design with future developments in dynamic reality.

The gamble may be a major one. The only available insurance against its magnitude is to be derived from a grand strategy that is complex and from specific strategies that are mutually complementary. The wager, when fully understood, is monumental. Its magnitude can be reduced only by the self-insurance of the philosopher and the inner assurance of the prophet. The philosopher's self-insurance has, in Kissinger's case, consisted in his pessimism regarding the West, which can be drawn upon to substantiate the limitations of even the most brilliant statecraft in averting deterioration. The prophet's assurance, which in Kissinger's case might rest on his implied optimism about the East, permits confidence in benign developments attributable to a combination of correct divination and the statesman's supreme daring in placing it at the basis of an essentially passive design. It is in this perspective, perhaps, that one might contemplate Kissinger's tendency to fluctuate, in function of practical successes and setbacks, between the two poles he himself had academically identified: the pole of the statesman and that of the prophet. If generalized prophecy is to substitute for grand strategy, however, and philosophic dualities are to relieve rather than compound policy dilemmas, it is proper for the prophet at this point of American history to delineate the future sharply and positively enough to either inspire or reassure. It is less fitting for him to seek and offer both refuge and solace in sterile prognostications of doom.

IV

In terms of yet another Kissingerian distinction, involving the interplay between genius and mediocrity in matters political, the drift from creative to routine diplomacy in Kissinger's later tenure raised questions to be faced by American foreign policy-makers in the future as well as by the eventual historian of the present as it becomes the past. Was the drift to routine the supremely self-sacrificing effort by Kissinger to clothe authentic greatness in the forms of mediocrity in order to adjust its policy product to a stable society's limited capacity to absorb genius? Or, alternatively, was Kissinger's endowment as creative diplomatic strategist such as to permit no more than the essentially mediocre imitation of greatness producing in due course institutionalized hysteria (in the form of congressional criticism and executive-legislative conflict on foreign policy) and, if not complete irresponsibility in Kissinger himself, then a tendency to avoid ultimate responsibility?[6]

Be it as it may, the Bismarckian type of statecraft initially transposed into U.S. foreign policy was limited in both real and immediately possible accomplishments. It was nonetheless the only currently available and historically tested method for even provisionally spanning the distance between the fundamentally constant end (to preserve an irreducible American position in the world) and the largely restricted means (for "imperial" or any other effective interventions in support of policy). The wide acceptance of the need to adjust somewhat the position and the even more thoroughgoing restriction on the range of readily available methods for doing so enhanced the impression of Kissinger's unprecedented facility to work diplomatic miracles through personal magic. As miracles became rarer, triumphs gave way to tribulations highlighting previously ignored flaws: superficially those of style and more seriously those of substance. Among the increasingly publicized flaws of style were secrecy, deception and duplicity, lack of compassion, and unprincipled opportunism. It was noted, among other things, that Kissinger inclined to lean toward the momentarily or tactically stronger party, be it the North Vietnamese, the Arabs, or the Turks, as a means first to acceptability as peacemaker and then to speedy if possibly short-lived accomplishments. Such flaws are offensive to what passes for indigenous American ethos, to be rescued once again from the corruption by foreign models. The indignation falls into place, however, when the critics of values eulogized Kissinger's mastery of diplomacy as unprecedented in American annals while the critics of the less attractive methods of activism from weakness were opposed to both neo-isolationism (the obverse of activism) and old-style imperialism (the obverse of weakness). Both kinds of critics helped, through their cooperation in stripping American foreign policy of effective instruments, to reduce Kissinger to the practice of diplomacy in its narrowest technical sense, which depends on skills along the condemned lines.

More serious was the feeling that, if Kissinger's statecraft lived

---

[6] The preceding query manipulates notions developed by Kissinger in his "The White Revolutionary: Reflections on Bismarck" in *Daedalus*, Summer 1968, pp. 888–90.

off the capital and credit built up in the cold-war or imperial era, it was unfolding outside any settled consensus about the future. The climate of revulsion arising from the Vietnam war permitted different political and economic concessions to the two Communist great powers to which previous administrations had been either unwilling or politically unable to consent. With the resurfacing of limits on continuing concessions, a marked slow-down occurred in the movement beyond stabilization to reconstruction, beyond relieving the world of anxieties toward restoring it on new foundations. In the area of conflict moderation, the initial successes in the Middle East owed much to the largely fortuitous local attitudes emerging from the latest war. But they were also due to encouraging the key country, Egypt, to expect substantial, imperial-style American economic and technological aid. The expectation was rooted in the American cold-war record and performance; it proved to be fallacious, as evenhandedness in diplomatic posture between the local contestants came to mean also empty-handedness in terms of foreign-policy instruments. The new situation had been foreshadowed in Southeast Asia, when the United States defaulted (at the first pretext) on its pledge to extend reconstruction aid to North Vietnam as part of the military agreement and as a prelude to political accommodation within Vietnam and between Hanoi and Washington.

Since a continuing draft on vanishing assets was certain to erode the American credit in the world beyond the capacity of anyone's personal credibility to make up for it, Kissinger could be criticized on this score only in the context of a corrective strategic conception. Instead of offering one, his critics tended to focus on deficiencies in the area of consensus. The absence of consensus on foreign policy to replace the one crystallized in the cold war and expired over Vietnam brought Kissinger one initial advantage. It facilitated the transition from the solidly equipped management of world order to an increasingly solitary diplomatic manipulation for regional peace. As the earlier consensus broke down, so did the related constraints on the making of foreign policy; but, for the same reason, the free hand for the diplomat abroad was matched by a free-for-all at home. Just about anyone in Congress and out could aspire to fill the doctrinal void and, in the process, share in replacing the fairly continuous foreign-policy élite which had dominated the scene between the Second World War and the second Indochina war. The advantage derived by the diplomat from his comparative freedom in dealing with foreign crises has thus been offset by the license which has found its way into domestic criticism likewise free of any serious constraint, including that implicit in the requirement for some internal coherence and consistency across issues. A diplomatic freedom so hampered is liable to be perverted, however, if consensus-free domestic pluralism intensifies the natural propensity of the manipulative, or Bismarckian, statesman to express himself through multi-purpose diplomacy—a diplomacy which calculates each and every major (and minor) step so as to make it serve several internal and external purposes at one and the same time.

In such conditions, the temptation is bound to be great for such a statesman to occasionally magnify crises in order to subsequently better manage them: to pass, in short, from the peace-at-hand stance to the war-in-sight posture. This will be especially true if the domestic power base of the maker of foreign policy has begun to weaken. Thus Kissinger was led, off and on, to dramatize the immediate risks of renewed fighting in the Middle East and the long-range dangers on the oil front in order to either magnify in perspective even token—but domestically increasingly essential—successes in appeasement or to protect his rear against charges of improvidence if catastrophe were to supervene. The price to pay for the indulgence seemed never to be too great. Thus, in connection with the economic and monetary crisis set off by the increase in oil price, Kissinger found it convenient to publicly revive fears of communization in Western Europe (Italy) in order to simultaneously impress anti-Communist (Saudi) oil-producers abroad and rehabilitate before liberal American opinion as enduringly useful the kind of clandestine measures the administration was being criticized for when applying them against the Allende regime. The voiced apprehensions may have been genuine and were well-founded up to a point; but the intensity and the timing of their public expression were, in the conditions of disintegrated consensus, subject to damaging hypothetical speculation about motives, speculation nourished by the kind of diplomatic rationality which is peculiar to the Bismarckian diplomatic artist himself and is quintessentially inseparable from him.

The simultaneous and reciprocally reinforcing erosion of foreign-policy consensus and domestic confidence in its personality surrogate will be especially fatal if the period of free hand has resulted in added national obligation arising out of semi-private understandings entered into as part of achieving success in peacemaking and mediation. Rightly or wrongly, rumors of such understandings and undertakings circulated in connection with both Indochina and the Middle East. In reintensified military crisis, the implicit commitments could not but depend for their fulfillment in either resource-expensive or risk-taking U.S. action on the abrupt reemergence of the very consensus whose absence made the American undertaking possible (by enlarging negotiating freedom) and necessary (by withholding alternative methods for securing the widely approved-of objective). Such an occasion would be the rude awakening from the earlier dream of cost-free accomplishments. It would test the solidity of the single-handed artifact in one or another geographic area; and it might stimulate a review of the nature and implications of the entire diplomatic system, not least toward bringing into a more stable relationship the ends and means of American foreign policy, by either scaling down the former or revitalizing the latter.

Whether or not valid in full or in large part, the foregoing observations about the Kissinger statecraft suggest both caveats and a higher form of criticism. First the caveats. On the issue of diplomatic style, Bismarckian manipulation or juggling was a flaw only when combined with Metternichian passion for caution: tactical ruthlessness with strategic timidity. If severed from a positive strategic object, the tactical Bismarckian arts become a rather lowly diplomatic form of *l'art pour l'art* in a void. The art is corruptive because not inherently creative and the artist overstates even false dangers because he fails to generate and assume the right kind of risks—risks that will substitute for deficient material resources in the short run while eliciting the needed resource from the domestic political system in the long run. If the Bismarckian style is denatured within a Metternichian substance, this will offend the democratic milieu in the name of its values without subjecting it to the bracing effect of a foreign policy requiring and deserving at least an intermittent degree of primacy over domestic politics. Freely manipulative diplomacy will then flourish only as long as democratic constraints on foreign-policy-making are temporarily suspended. It will fail to consolidate the domestic leeway with a flexible balance of power system abroad—i.e., with the aid of the very workings of the latter and its hard-to-dispute requirements.

The most recent congressional revolt against executive leeway in foreign policy has found expression in both specific inhibitions and procedural constraints, notably on the use of force abroad. Pushed to the extreme, the legislators' insurgence against past policies and mistrust of current policymaking threatened to create a new kind of danger, however, even as Congress sought to eliminate the risk of future abuses. The danger was one of actually forcing the policymaker into escalating crisis situations to a pitch sufficient to free him from low-level congressional inhibitions (e.g., on aid to foreign countries under congressional cloud, such as Turkey) or to induce the Congress itself to exercise its newly reasserted powers (over the use of force) in conformity with the executive's perception of foreign-policy requirements.[7] Any such compulsion on the executive, passed on by him to the Congress, would erode an important restraint that was operative throughout the cold-war period. The executive was then free to engage in verbal escalation when describing outside threats in order to secure congressional cooperation—e.g., prior to the enactment of the Truman and Eisenhower doctrines. But the restraint militated against actually intensifying a crisis by deeds of omission or commission—such as may have preceded Pearl Harbor, according to one interpretation of that concluding event of the isolationist era.

When the Congress fosters a situation reducing the executive to a more or less subtle manufacture of crises, it can not protect itself effectively against the unintended consequence as long as it is unable, by its nature, to monitor every important diplomatic maneuver or other occurrence that might lead to a crisis within a flexible international system and related diplomatic system. Any such in-

---

[7] Since the above was written, the Mayagüez incident in the Bay of Siam off Cambodia has displayed aspects substantiating the above proposition, if on a (characteristically) minor scale. The element of deliberate crisis escalation was, however, probably more authentic than had been demonstrably the case for the Gulf of Tonkin incident off North Vietnam occurring in an earlier and qualitatively different era.

ability reduces to a fiction, however, the Congress' specifically inhibitory capacity and broadly procedural powers bearing on the use of force, and it weakens its overall supervisory role in foreign policy. The foreign policy of diplomatic maneuver differs in two essential respects from the cold-war and imperial foreign policy of management. To begin with, the possibility of legislative-executive conflict in the latter was minimized by a strong foreign-policy consensus reflecting a widely shared feeling of insecurity which favored congressional acceptance of executive leadership in foreign affairs. More to the point, occasion for inter-branch conflict was reduced also by the fact that the instruments of foreign policy over which the Congress habitually exercises its strongest power of appropriations, such as national armaments and foreign economic and military aid, were more than the essence of foreign policy. In conditions of settled foreign-policy challenges and objectives, the instruments were, in effect, coterminous with the substance of foreign policy most of the time. This fact alone guaranteed executive concern for coordination with the legislative branch as effectively as the insecurity environment insured legislative compliance with major executive initiatives.

In the situation now emerging, salience has been shifting to economic issues (with high domestic implications) *pari passu* with reductions in politico-military insecurity; but, at least in the short run and despite overlaps, diplomatic maneuvers are also more readily distinguishable and separable from economic and financial issues than was world-order management, American style. The result has been a new tension between a latent and freshly significant weakness of the Congress (as an organ unsuited to day-by-day monitoring of the nuances of diplomatic maneuver) and its real strength (to apply its control over the nation's purse in ways attuned to internal group pressures) apparently enhanced by the proliferation of foreign-policy issues with high economic component. It is to this tension that one must look for pressures to restore executive-legislative harmony on broad substance of foreign policy as well as on the procedures of foreign-policy-making that would incorporate adequate executive autonomy along with both responsiveness and responsibility. Such autonomy is necessary for manipulative balance-of-power diplomacy. It will be also required to shield the American constitutional system and political culture from the ambiguities of deliberate crisis-escalation in the well-intentioned service of the national interest.

A style and methods of manipulative diplomacy that were denatured as part of a strategically too-cautious or insufficiently productive diplomacy helped engender reactive parliamentary constraints and might aggravate, as an ulterior consequence, an "irresponsibly" risk- and crisis-maximizing foreign policy. In addition to a malproportioned tactical-strategic relationship, there is yet another reason why the proper relationship between democratic consensus and the diplomatist's free hand can be deranged, with resulting distortion and eventual erosion of the latitude that is required by both specifically Bismarckian and generally balancing strategy. Such a derangement is liable to take place when the exercise of inspired statecraft turns into its public exhibition and procedurally "free" hand into an unnecessary personalization of substantive foreign policies. In a democratic milieu highly amenable to the metamorphosis, a desirable measure of insulation of foreign policy from domestic politics is then sooner or later victimized by the identification between policy and the incumbent policymaker. This will make foreign policy unduly dependent on the statesman's domestic political fortunes while making the statesman himself the captive of his policies in relation to the foreign powers on which the success of the strategy (and thus his own success) may well come to depend. Personalization of policies will thus either distort or reduce the flexibility required for the international equilibrium system; and it may be prejudicial to the domestic system of checks and balances. That is to say, highly personalized policymaking will engender a bias in favor of strategies which, by evolving gradually over time, make the originating policymaker indispensable (for securing an ever-receding consummation and dealing with ever-deferred contingencies, including confrontations) while permitting him to be non-responsible along the ever-lengthening line between the policy's origination and its outcome. The more the long-term policies degenerate into routine diplomacy and incur the dangers of immobilization, the likelier is the evolution of the domestic free hand into foreign captivity. Such as it is, this danger does not warrant confining the Bismarckian statesman in either a finely articulated domestic consensus concerning details of substantive foreign policy or a crudely structured parliamentary control over the procedures of its executive implementation. It does justify, however, a close inspection of the statesman's personal and, indeed, professional ethos, including his readiness for impersonal subordination to an ideal standard of public service. Such an ethos is independent of the specific, democratic or other, values and convictions that are deemed incompatible with free-handed equilibrium statecraft while being all too often but self-congratulatory civic myths with scarce relevance for foreign policy.

A truly serious value question arises only in connection with the issue of justice or equity. However, just as the balance-of-power process nearly automatically crystallizes an interstate consensus about its rules, so the counterpoising of conflicting interests and values tends to administer rough substantive justice or equity. It will do so, within the practically attainable limits, in excess of the reliable measure of such justice emanating from even an enlightened single power holder. This is the deeper meaning of the notion of the "just equilibrium," supplemental to its ritualistic significance and invocative usage. It will be inevitable that, in the process of allocating rough substantive justice through the equilibrium mechanism, even salient individual interests will be sacrificed, and with them, occasionally and then dramatically, justice for one or more parties. But it is not for a political society such as America's, reared on the principle of both constitutional and social and political checks and balances, to question—or reject as incompatible with its internal value system—the nearest international equivalent of its own dominant guarantor of approximate equity: not, that is, unless it is also prepared to surrender itself internally to either enlightened despotism or politically unredeemed constitutional judicialism. To see "justice" as emanating at least in part from equilibrium is a necessary corrective to the tendency—manifest in Kissinger, among others, when discoursing on the subject in his idealized Metternichian vein—to differentiate equilibrium and justice (or agreement on what constitutes justice) as two separate and equivalent factors in and for both spontaneous stability and supple negotiation. In actuality, what is regarded as "just" and "fair" in any particular case of contention short of direct physical coercion will be, in relative terms, more a reflection of the distribution of power than that distribution in general and over time is a function of the inherent justice—or capacity for abstract justice—of the political societies which make up the equilibrium situation.

A different set of considerations is prompted by the issue of concessions from the American cold war capital. If a free hand must be constrained from within by the statesman's rigid ethos of service and the demand for societal and parliamentary consensus constrained from without by the efficacy requirements of a flexible equilibrium strategy, the granting or denying of concessions must be governed by the provision for compensation. The issue is not whether concessions are of tangible or intangible assets, extensive or limited, sudden or gradual—or even whether they are offset by individual counter-concessions in a particular context. What matters is whether the surrender of assets accumulated in one constellation can be compensated with systemically guaranteed certainty over time in the constellation which their surrender has helped to bring into being. The fact that the Western European democracies, when embarking in the 1930s on appeasement from a superior initial position but not from intrinsic strength, failed to employ and apportion the concessions consented to Germany efficiently enough to rebalance the international system in new dimensions neither discredits nor foredooms such strategy in the 1970s. The United States of today is even less the Britain of 1938 than it is the Britain of 1900. As the international system is enlarged—in its diplomatically active geopolitical space and in its structural and, consequently, functional diversity—the previously impossible concessions become possible even as the previously vital assets become irrelevant.

Along with the issues raised by the risk-resource tradeoff, the issue highlighted by the inquiry into what constitutes tolerable concessions is the prime basis for a higher Kissinger criticism. It does not revolve around the question of the degree of concession from the cold war asset pile, but around the degree of continuing consummation or consolidation of the post–cold war or post-imperial international system; not around the issue of tactical juggling or deceiving, but around the question of the expended effort and achieved success in interrelating détente and devolution strategies, great and lesser-power hierarchies and levels, and *ad hoc* conflict and concert in and for different regions in a grand, Bismarckian strategy for leadership in equilibrium politics. Such higher criticism suggests some major propositions. The Bismarckian system as adumbrated by the Nixon-Kissinger team was either a serious undertaking, and then ought to have been pursued, or was an opportunistic device for momentary relief (in Vietnam) and pressure (on the Soviets), and then did not deserve the importance attributed to it; moreover, if the triangular diplomatic system is not developed it is apt to deteriorate into conditions worse than those antecedent to it. Another, related proposition is that the alternative conservative or Metternichian design was premature for America's stage as both a power and a society, while being potentially productive of what it postulates: external decline and internal demoralization, redressible *in extremis* by a calamitous diplomatic revolution from weakness if at all. Further, if the prevalent diplomatic system was intended as a compromise between the Bismarckian, the Metternichian, and a truncated or residual imperial system, then the synthesis has been either lopsided in favor of the Metternichian strain or amorphous to the point where the component parts become indistinguishable and might be reciprocally nullifying in intended or possible effect. This is so mainly because both the proximate strategic objective and the identity of the clarified terminal diplomatic system have been impressed with an ambiguity so great as to induce and warrant anonymity.

From such major propositions can be derived a few minor or subsidiary ones. They suggest that Kissinger may have confounded philosophic doctrine with diplomatic strategy to the detriment of the latter. This would explain his launching an essentially simple conservative design without an adequate support from a sustaining complex strategy, as distinct from an elaborate tactical apparatus. By trying to conserve the principal inherited assets, he failed to move far and fast enough to consolidate a more viable new system of alignments. He lost thus a rare occasion, offered by the exceptional post-Vietnam latitude within the United States and receptiveness outside it, for reorienting American foreign policy from empire to equilibrium while retaining for it a leadership role. In a similar way, if perhaps with more reason, his predecessors had lost the opportunity offered by the Vietnam war to implant an imperial role as maintainer of world order in the public's minds and loyalties. Finally, by responding to the reduction of available material and political resources for a directly "costly" foreign (or imperial) policy, he failed to recognize the need for compensation in the area of assumed risks in order to increase the long-term prospects for preserving essential U.S. interests by virtue of reshaping the international system in more dimensions than are encompassed by the unquestionably salient, but not solely important, U.S.-Soviet relations.

The critique, while sweepingly systemic, appeared to be not altogether academic at a time that exhibited little perceptible unfolding of the Kissingerian conservative grand design, as the sequence to the previously abandoned Kennedyite design of the liberal *grand empire*. This was also the time when, in the lowlands of the lesser-state turmoils, neither intervention nor linkages were in evidence and when the small steps of mediatory diplomacy in the Middle East depended, instead, on the continuance of exceptionally propitious local circumstances, while the peacemaker was indisposed to retrace the wearying path toward political settlement in Southeast Asia amid military setbacks.

As it gradually subsided into manifest slowdown and possible impasse, the post-Vietnam diplomacy identified with Kissinger was increasingly reminiscent of the post-Algerian diplomacy of Charles de Gaulle, the most contemporary model of both Nixon and Kissinger. It is possible to take into account differences in the intentions inspiring the statecraft of the Frenchman and of the Americans, not least with respect to Western Europe, as well as the differences in national material base. The first difference supplies an extenuating circumstance, while the second is an aggravating one when measuring Kissinger's attainments against de Gaulle's. So adjusted, the fact remains that neither will have recast the relations between the United States and Western Europe on the basis of either effective unilateral leadership or effective bilateral relations in such a way as to set in motion a discernible European evolution over time into a systemic counterpart to China. And both failed to recast relations with China sufficiently to move the Soviet Union to a meaningfully adaptive response. From de Gaulle's viewpoint, this meant making the Soviets accept France-in-Western Europe as the valid interlocutor in entente diplomacy (relative to the United States); for the United States, it meant operationalizing détente and changes toward approximate parity in ways consistent with overall American equilibrium leadership in areas outside highly abstract (nuclear) or highly materialistic (trade-cum-technology) issues. In his attempts, de Gaulle was largely baffled by American opposition and Soviet opportunism. Both fed into the intra-European resistance to great or small changes if those changes were to enhance French "grandeur" even symbolically. In the end, de Gaulle was defeated by the overall shapelessness of the American policies, focused on Vietnam, in the period following Kennedy's rival grand design; even American contrariness was then lacking as the spring that might lift French diplomacy above the level of its inherent leverage. A similar indeterminacy has since threatened to overcome Kissinger's design as he moved, still in de Gaulle's steps in the post-heroic phase, into the only superficially dramatic diplomacy of itinerant statecraft punctuated with stillborn grand designs for different continents and international organizations. There has even been, though differently for Kissinger than for de Gaulle, a growing inclination to escape from diplomatic frustrations into economic (or economically relevant) realizations, less in response to the weight of past criticisms than as a tribute to the lightening of both personal and national weight in the scales wherein everything else must in the end repose.

De Gaulle's prophetic quality as seer of needs and trends redeemed the frustrations thwarting his statecraft. Can or will the same lot befall Kissinger's? There have been many who were anxious to undertake the demonstration that Kissinger's traditionalist balance-of-power approach was obsolete for a world that must not be restored if it is to be transformed to implement transnational interdependence. The slowdown in creative diplomacy will seemingly vindicate this kind of criticism. It has been, therefore, more appropriate for a commentary conceived in terms of reference basically akin to Kissinger's own to suggest that his performance might have been as much at fault as his premises. That is to say, he applied the balance-of-power method incompletely in one respect and prematurely in another: incompletely, because he applied it in the last resort only to the Soviet Union as part of a revision or inversion of antagonistic bipolarity; and, therefore, prematurely, in that the transition from antagonism to accommodation has occurred before devolution elsewhere had activated—or begun to activate—supplementary leverages on Soviet conduct and

structural reinsurance against the failure of U.S.-Soviet conciliation. To this contention must be opposed the previously examined
one that a fuller multi-power equilibrium policy would have been
either anachronistic (because coming too late) or premature (because being instituted in full too early). Either of the diagnoses
can be validly argued in terms of the concepts and norms of traditional statecraft. All differ radically and, from the traditionalist
viewpoint, favorably from contentions indicting Kissinger's statecraft with being obsolete in basic conception, in that it downplayed
economics for politics and environmental issues for equilibrium. It
is possible to reverse the charge of obsolescence. The basic argument behind the charge has been that while the management and
configuration of politico-military power was rightfully the prime
need in the period following World War II, the passing of the cold
war has transferred primacy to economic and related issues both
nationally and internationally in conformity with changes in the
nature of the dual—domestic and global—crisis. An opposing
argument would contend, however, that while the structure of
power and conflict was basically determined in the earlier instance
by the course and outcome of the war, its fluid and uncrystallized
transitional character has recently required all the more attention.
To manage power is not only to enact and survive polarized conflict: it is also, and more demandingly, to shape configurations so
as to economize on force by dispersing both power and conflicts.

To this may be added a final caveat. It is the proper use of the
endowments and energies of the international statesman to try to
influence both global and regional balances of power so as to make
their dynamic impede adverse economic combinations of lesser
powers and counteract the economic intrigues of the greater ones.
Being proper, that use is also more economical than use in the
attempt to directly shape the international distribution of welfare
or directly influence a nation's balance of trade. The supreme
anachronism for an actually or potentially neo-mercantilist world
is *not* to disinter eighteenth-century statecraft. It is to revive a mid-
nineteenth-century ideology, thus pretending to divorce political
power from economics internationally—or, now, "transnation-
ally." Major objectives, from American-Soviet détente to the unity
of Europe or Germany, may be pursued by the economic road
without much chance for conclusive progress beyond an indeter-

minate middle zone defined by recurrent partial advances and re-
treats and by reciprocally frustrating competition over special
advantages or "special relationships." The limitations of the *Zoll-
verein* strategy[8] are liable to restore in due course the attractions
of the Bismarckian strategy. When this occurs, the prior inversion
of the classic liberal separation of economics and politics into the
identification of economics with high policy in an internally falter-
ing and externally (apparently) secure semi-liberal economic system may once again collapse, yielding to the primacy of the authentic high policy with military-strategic overtones. In the
contemporary setting, "real" politics may become ascendant again
in the context of either internal reactions to deepening economic
deterioration in the West (and in Japan) or of external revisions
sought on the basis of internally growing economic capabilities by
the powers of the Communist East. As long as such longer-term
evolutions cannot be ruled out, it is safer for the nation's interests
—and incumbent upon its stewards—to be obsolescent if the alternative is to be utopian, just as it is imperative at critical turning
points to be forceful if the alternative is to be irresolutely fabian.

---

[8] I.e., attempts to promote German unity through customs union in the
earlier nineteenth century.

VI. KISSINGER: APPRAISALS AND ALTERNATIVES

Viewed in a demanding perspective, Kissinger's statecraft does not rate exceptionally high. Outside a perspective, it has proven difficult to go beyond chicanery about Kissinger's style (including his penchant for transactions with authoritarian adversaries) and his inconsistencies as statesman and as scholar (involving the treatment of allies). The difficulty, which was manifest during most of Kissinger's official tenure, has been an unwitting tribute to the elusiveness of the subject, i.e., is his lack of consistent drive toward a definable achievement either in relations with the great powers or in relations among the lesser powers. There has been little to tear down critically since, beyond global "normalization," so little has been built or consolidated that has gone beyond overall appeasement. That appeasement, moreover, reflected a stage in the cycle of waxing and waning conflict long overdue by any standard based on historical precedents for the post–World War II era. To note the fact that Kissinger's philosophic commitment to repose or restoration fitted the times is not to prove that it was Kissinger's statecraft that appeased the world. It may be more correct to suggest that Kissinger's philosophical commitment inhibited him from efforts that might have exploited the basic inclination of the major Communist powers for aiming at policy results that would—or could, at risk—convert the inclination into more irreversible consummations and commitments than those apparently secured. In appearances at least, Kissinger alternated between the posture of philosopher (high priest of repose and prophet of doom?) and tactically or routinely oriented diplomatist (bargainer and concession-broker), avoiding the all-important intermediate area of constellating strategy most of the time.

A lack of architectonic dimension in the design of Kissingerian diplomacy, and of continuity across issues in its execution, was reflected in what was previously identified as "shuttle diplomacy" in a broader-than-usual meaning of the term. To move from issue to issue is fundamentally different from projecting issue against issue in a multi-faceted diplomatic system—or, differently put, in a system-wide diplomacy. Even the linkage diplomacy as advertised at the beginning of the Nixon administration is conceptually but an elementary variety of juggling issues while counterpoising powers against one another. Such juggling is the necessary manipulative counterpart to in-depth managerial efforts at equilibration of capabilities, to be carried out on the level where seizable handles to underlying processes are in existence. If Kissinger did juggle, his manipulation involved the immediate parties to a specific issue in terms of selective personal communications, disclosures, and commitments only. Little of the more difficult juggling across issues and regions was in evidence, and it was most conspicuously absent from the peacemaking for the Middle East and Southeast Asia. Similarly, if Kissinger played a "hard game" in bureaucratic infighting and interallied contentions, and if he occasionally may have played such a game with adversaries (when unilateralizing Middle Eastern peacemaking with an ostensible anti-Soviet bias or when threatening to "link" this or that with détente), it does not necessarily means that he was not timid strategically at the same time.

Kissinger has loomed large for contemporaries as both statesman and personality. But, paradoxically, it is more than commonly possible in his case to differentiate the realizations of American foreign policy and his uniquely personal contribution to them. American foreign policy was relatively successful in the period coinciding with the first six years or so of Kissinger's official tenure, considering the context and the limitations under which it labored. No immediately catastrophic or, if a reversal from late-Kissingerian trends occurs in time, manifestly irreversible deterioration in the American position took place while great-power relations were being superficially stabilized. At the same time, the main components of the adopted policy were more self-evident and virtually self-executing than is habitual for periods covering the break with one mold (cold war/imperial) and the transition to a different one. The Communist great powers were manifestly ready to go through a phase of moderation and accommodation. Intimations from the Soviet Union were not lacking, and it was a signal from the Chinese themselves of their readiness to "normalize" relations with the United States that apparently set off the implementation of a process—or, at least, the first steps in a process—that was henceforth desired by both sides. Only a full knowledge of what transpired, of the undertakings and understandings entered into, would permit a sure judgment on whether the price paid (over and beyond that implicit in Nixon's pilgrimage to Peking) was excessive relative to the secured benefits—indeed, whether the pledged reparation for past American sins was not too extensive to be actually made in anything like a policy-relevant time span and was not thus a too onerous charge on developing relations in the future. If the Communist powers were ready for appeasement, moreover, the shell-shocked American public was even more so. And there were no perceptible impediments in the international environment, such as effectively resistant allies in either of the great-power camps or a Third World anxious to forestall and capable of hindering movement away from the easily exploitable American-Soviet bipolarity of the cold war era.

If there is any truth in the preceding remarks, Kissinger's extra contribution to restructuring relations among the great powers can be safely discounted below the level of contemporary acclaim. There is, beyond that, no present way to evaluate his skills as negotiator with the north Vietnamese and the distinctive contribution these skills made even within the limited scope of the military disengagement alone. It is possible to hazard the general view that the ongoing rearrangement of inter-great power relations and the reprieve that American foreign policy gained by the mere transfer of presidential powers for Vietnamization and for the application of very specific military measures were more important than any personal ascendancy in negotiating with adversaries of the caliber of the North Vietnamese. The positive change in the overall strategic environment must be attributed to Nixon himself, however, as regards immediate agency (i.e., the fact and circumstances of being elected) and ultimate responsibility and risk (i.e., his continuing liability to electoral sanction). Pending contrary evidence, furthermore, it is possible to attribute to the former president the fundamental strategic conceptions as well. In this respect, the theses publicized by the two principals before acquiring the official base for action will remain a useful source for equitable distribution of merit to contrast with post-event reconstitutions by principals and proxies alike.

136

The next and more important question is: While making his great or not-so-great personal contribution, was Kissinger a climactic figure or only a transitional one? And, in either case, did he demonstrate the continuing existence of a significant latitude for individual achievement in international politics in a democracy, or did he not? Kissinger would emerge as a climactic figure if it came to appear that his tenure coincided, to say the least, with the consummation of a drawn-out evolution of American foreign policy toward maturity as a great power among great powers. Such maturity means correctly measuring feasible goals and husbanding means for their attainment within the limits set by both domestic and external claims on the means and challenges to the goals. One might then judge that, in such a perspective, it was both justified and provident to avoid immediately unnecessary risks and to concentrate mainly on gaining time—both globally and on regional peace issues—for promising political trends to materialize, transient economic dislocations to be moderated, and relations to be routinized "spontaneously." Kissinger's prudent statecraft, his self-limitation to bargaining over small-state issues and to a combination of concessionary nuclear strategy and largely ceremonial interpersonal diplomacy over superpower issues with but rare and symbolic evocation of force (e.g., naval movements and nuclear alert), would then be vindicated by the rightness of Kissinger's philosophic perception of needs and trends even while being considered too much of a wager in the light of more skeptical philosophy and too little of a gamble in a more exacting strategic perspective. The only problem would then be how to reconcile Kissinger's philosophic optimism, implicit in the mere nursing of postulated favorable trends vis-à-vis the "East," and the philosophic pessimism that informed his public broodings over the social and political debilities of the West.

Conversely Kissinger may appear as only a transitional figure, a caretaker rather than a creator, between two distinctive major phases of American foreign policy and two unevenly homogeneous foreign policy élites. This would be the case for policy if Kissinger's tenure as secretary of state were to deteriorate into self-serving operations terminating in reintensified regional and systemic crises calling for philosophically more tentative and strategically more determinate and determined responses—responses, that is, that would either remobilize the necessary resources and disposition for a more vigorous American self-assertion or else crystallize into policy the mood of national self-abandonment. It would not much matter then whether Kissinger's approach was condemned retrospectively (with different degrees of justice for reasons unevenly of Kissinger's making) as either primarily mismanaged or primarily misconceived. More importantly, the entire Nixon-Kissinger-Ford era would then appear as having been but a holding operation between the exertions of action (cold war and Vietnam) and the exertions of response (to the world as it "really" was after Vietnam)—as a breathing spell afforded by the transient restraint of the Communist powers and the temporary retreat of alternative or rival élites at home.

The latitude due to the élite vacuum followed from a certain moral dissolution of the preceding foreign-policy élite and the only incipient re-formation of a successor élite. The composition or profile of the successor élite in the future will depend on the evolving setting of policy. Even the semblance of a Kissinger failure—be it "absolute" or relative to the cultivated image of the miracleworker—may partially rehabilitate the remainders or offshoots of the "Brahmin" élite that had been discredited in different circles either by its sliding into, or by its wobbling over, Vietnam. Watergate has already partially rehabilitated that élite by default. It compared favorably, in terms of presumed individual and collective integrity, with the Nixon brand of surrogate élite deriving from more varied or less assured social, ethnic, and (domestically) regional backgrounds. The trend to rehabilitation would accelerate if the post-Kissinger environment also favored greater individual and collective self-effacement and, conjointly, greater dependence on procedural mechanisms rather than types of substantive policy for minimizing individual risk and responsibility. If, furthermore, developments restored validity to either the cold war or the imperial modes that had culminated in the military engagement in Southeast Asia, this might vindicate the traditional élite's basic and original judgments; or, alternatively, the same set of events might favor an ethnically and socially less uniform fresh élite, less demonstrably indisposed to hold to a course in adversity than had been the "Anglo-Saxon" managers of the national portfolio from the Eastern seaboard. Finally, the nature of the crisis and of the related capacity requirements might turn away from managing politico-military confrontations to competitively managing the "ties" of economic interdependence. This, too, would affect the criteria of eligibility for élite function and status in some degree.

In either case, Kissinger would loom as a figure of transition: allowed to step into the momentary élite vacuum under the auspices of a non-Establishment president; subsequently tolerated while carrying out the awkward liquidation or reduction of empire; and finally disowned as a mixture of fraud and failure—as had been Nixon himself—when the task was finished in depth and the performance faltered on the surface—an American Alberoni[1] rather than an American Bismarck. If the successor élite were to take over in the environment of a primarily economic crisis, it could be expected to reemphasize the traditional bias of U.S. foreign policy in favor of a high organizational component, regardless of whether the foreign-policy élite itself was or was not leavened with old-Establishment elements. It would probably replace diplomatic maneuver with organizational-functional gimmicks, just as diplomatic maneuver followed upon imperial management.

Independent of its ultimate success or failure, Kissinger's tenure and performance will have redirected attention to the latitude that a single—and, in some ways, strong—personality can sometimes enjoy in the shaping and conduct of foreign policy in a representative democracy. That latitude had been initially Nixon's, and it reflected his work style; its continuance was due to the paralysis of government and public fixation on one issue attending Watergate. More basically, however, that latitude was the function of the transition itself from the cold-war/imperial to some subsequent more settled or institutionalized diplomatic and international systems. As the cake of custom—or substantive consensus—crumbled, there was a greater leeway for individualistic or idiosyncratic foreign policy, just as the simultaneous élite vacuum created room at the top for one who, despite extended past associations, was in more normal conditions still essentially an outsider to be "on tap but not on top." That exceptional opening could be

---

[1] Foreign-born Alberoni was one of the more ambitious and briefly successful foreign ministers of declining Spain under the new Bourbon dynasty in the early eighteenth century.

enlarged and consolidated only by real, visible, and not automatically self-perpetuating achievement in foreign policy. It could be only temporarily kept open by diplomatic pyrotechnics and by a type of personality whose very difference from the predominant indigenous mold would either dazzle or antagonize—and actually did both in succession. When serious setbacks followed upon superficial successes, the margin for individuality began to narrow. Institutional constraint began to close in, at first mainly in terms of oppositional congressional obstruction without much internal coherence and criticism without much substantive content. Kissinger had been propelled to the heights by the recoil of the American political class (and mass) from the norm of bureaucratic—and, if not bureaucratic, then at least collective—foreign-policy making that was suspected of having incrementally led the nation into the Vietnam quagmire. By the same token, Kissinger became increasingly vulnerable to the desire for returning to normalcy in recoil from the nervous strain of individual hero-worship.

It is important for the foreign-policy scholar to determine whether Kissinger utilized the interlude of freedom from domestic constraints to the full and for the best; it was for the preceding discussion to attempt a delineation of the framework for such judgment. Beyond that, it is for the sociologist to determine what kind of hero-figure is most likely to last in the media-saturated American political culture feeding alternately on the build-up of the hero and on his demotion. Nor ought it to be without interest for the student of American society, even one hardened to the need for simplifying foreign-policy phenomena for public consumption, to examine and contrast the exaltation of Kissinger's works and the excoriation of his methods; the fascination with style as compared with substance; and the ways in which the theater of summits and pontifical summations outshone the drama of high policy caught up in the issues of national growth and decline.

BIBLIOGRAPHICAL NOTE

Sir Harold Nicolson's *Diplomacy* (New York: Oxford University Press, 1963) remains the standard short work on diplomacy and diplomatic styles. The history of the modern European state-system is masterfully summarized by the German historian Ranke in his essay on "The Great Powers" (printed in English translation in Theodore H. Von Laue, *Leopold Ranke: The Formative Years* [Princeton: Princeton University Press, 1950]) and, writing in the same tradition, by Ludwig Dehio in *The Precarious Balance* (New York: Knopf, 1962).

The diplomatic system of Wenzel Anton von Kaunitz-Rietberg, and its larger setting, can be explored in Walter L. Dorn, *Competition for Empire, 1740–1763* (New York: Harper and Row, 1940, 1963) and in M. S. Anderson, *Europe in the Eighteenth Century, 1713–1783* (London: Longmans, Green, 1961). Edward Crankshaw's *Maria Theresa* (New York: Viking Press, 1970) is both readable and anti-Kaunitz.

Kissinger's highly favorable view of Klemens von Metternich and his statecraft, reflecting the modern reappraisal of the Austrian statesman by Heinrich von Srbik, is enshrined in *A World Restored: Metternich, Castlereagh, and the Problem of Peace, 1812–22* (Boston: Houghton Mifflin, 1957). Metternich is less central and impressive to historians of the Congress of Vienna and the European Concert inclining to a different protagonist (Lord Castlereagh, in C. K. Webster's *The Foreign Policy of Castlereagh,* 2 vols.; Tsar Alexander, in W. A. Phillips, *The Confederation of Europe*; and Talleyrand, in G. Ferrero, *The Reconstruction of Europe*). Balanced treatments of Metternich and his era are found in Arthur J. May, *The Age of Metternich, 1814–1848* (New York: Holt, Rinehart, and Winston, 1963) and Guillaume de Bertier de Sauvigny, *Metternich and his Times* (London: Darton, Longman and Todd, 1962).

A convenient introduction to the Bismarck controversy is found in Thedore S. Hameron, ed., *Otto von Bismarck: A Historical Assessment* (Lexington, Mass.: Heath, 1972). Henry A. Kissinger discusses Bismarck and compares him (both implicitly and unfavorably) with Metternich in "The White Revolutionary: Reflections on Bismarck" (*Daedalus*, vol. 97, nos. 3–4 [Summer 1968]). An extensive and sympathetic discussion of Bismarck's diplomacy after 1870 is to be found in William L. Langer's *European Alliances and Alignments 1871–1890* (New York: Knopf, 1962). By contrast, A. J. P. Taylor is critical in both *Bismarck: The Man and the Statesman* (London: Hamish Hamilton, 1955) and *The Struggle for Mastery in Europe 1848–1918* (Oxford: Clarendon Press, 1954). A classic biography from the liberal viewpoint is Erich Eyck's *Bismarck and the German Empire* (London: Allen and Unwin, 1955).

Among the illuminating detailed accounts of early-eighteenth- and mid-nineteenth-century diplomacy worth noting are Basil Williams, *Stanhope: A Study in Eighteenth-Century War and Diplomacy* (Oxford: Clarendon Press, 1932, 1968); Sir Richard Lodge, *Studies in Eighteenth-Century Diplomacy 1740–1748* (London: J. Murray, 1930), and G. B. Henderson, *Crimean War Diplomacy and other Historical Essays* (Glasgow: Jackson, 1947). The ideas behind classic statecraft are explored by Friedrich Meinecke in *Machiavellism: The Doctrine of Raison d'Etat and Its Place in Modern History* (New York: Praeger, 1965).

Academic criticism of the basic premises of Kissinger's "traditionalist" statecraft by international-relations scholars of note, including Stanley Hoffmann and Zbigniew Brzezinski, can be found in past issues of the quarterlies *Foreign Affairs* and *Foreign Policy*. One of the journalistic Kissinger-watchers and regular traveling companions, Marvin L. Kalb, has produced in *Kissinger* a close-up of the subject (Boston: Little, Brown, 1974), which ought to humanize austere academic treatments.

APPENDIX*
A GUARANTEE FOR ISRAEL

I

With Secretary Kissinger's return from his Middle Eastern mission, a sudden urgency was injected into the issue of a U.S. security guarantee to Israel or Israel and Egypt jointly, to the accompaniment of trial balloons and official denials concerning the all-important question of whether what is to be guaranteed is an interim Israeli-Egyptian agreement now or only a final settlement eventually. Only a day or two after Kissinger's return, James Reston of the *Times*[1] has come out in support of a U.S. guarantee of secure and recognized 1967 borders, after rehearsing standing contrary arguments (i.e., the danger of Soviet counter-guarantees and different degrees of Arab and European disgruntlement) that make sense only if an American guarantee were to precede or replace a settlement. Misled or misleading, Reston's plaidoyer followed an open one by Richard Ullman, Director of Studies at the Council on Foreign Relations, in the January 1975 issue of *Foreign Affairs*.[2]

* The text which makes up the Appendix was originally written by prearrangement for a weekly magazine of opinion, within days after Secretary of State Kissinger's return from his exploratory mission to the Middle East in late February 1975, preliminary to its abortive continuance in March. While the article was being prepared and submitted, the issue of an interim U.S. guarantee evaporated under authoritative denials from State Department spokesmen. Much of the argument thus lost immediate relevance and the article was not published. I reprint the text here virtually verbatim in the hope that some of the points going beyond the issue of an interim guarantee will be helpful in concretizing the more general statements advanced in the principal text in relation to the Middle East. It may enhance the reader's sense of possible future relevance of the guarantee issue, as well, if he mentally substitutes a term such as "informal assurances" for the term "guarantee," and "restatement" (of the informal American guarantee) for (its) "formalization," with respect to situations anterior to a final political settlement in the area.

[1] "Guarantee for Israel?," *New York Times*, February 21, 1975, p. 31.
[2] "After Rabat: Middle East Risks and American Roles," pp. 284–96.

143

Ullman argues for a U.S. guarantee as one that, accompanied by Israeli withdrawals, would help lay "the foundation for a long-term settlement" and deter the next war on or by Israel. Complementing Reston's column, moreover, inspired Egyptian leaks, Israeli interpretations and imputations, and an unattributed State Department denial have been sufficiently contradictory to confuse without convincing. It is thus both immediately hazardous and preventively useful to raise the question of whether an interim guarantee would be a good thing for the United States, for a long-term Middle Eastern settlement, and for Israel itself, in that order.

A U.S. guarantee to both Israel and Egypt (an idea bruited about by the Egyptians) would amount to a Middle Eastern Locarno. The original was Britain's (and Italy's) guarantee of France and Germany against one another's aggression in the 1920s. Any interposition of neutral or U.S. or superpower forces would back up the Locarno formula with a human Maginot line facing both ways. Nearly everybody in the West, including the Europeans, is agreed that something along these lines is required to stabilize an eventual political settlement. Why, then, the sudden dramatization which, by anticipating such settlement, risks antagonizing the non-Egyptian Arab parties while stirring up a hornet's nest in this country? When the issue of guaranteeing the political settlement becomes acute, moreover, it will not be a Soviet counter-guarantee but a Soviet co-guarantee or parallel guarantee that will be pertinent. It is of questionable diplomatic taste to appear to be prejudging the issue unilaterally, just when we are shifting both diplomatic gears and hopes for peace from the unilateral step-by-step approach toward a common superpower approach. Nor does it make compelling sense to agitate the U.S. guarantee issue now in order to gain diplomatic leverage from a congressionally certified ability of the United States to institute peace in the Middle East unilaterally (after failing to so negotiate it) by linking the guarantee to a one-step total Israeli withdrawal. This would amount to a *de facto* anti-Israel settlement, notably on the West Bank, without any compensation outside the redundant formalization of the American commitment.

Reasoning along these lines imparts greater plausibility to the unofficial Egyptian version, as against the State Department's, as to what is being considered, if not readied. It furthermore imparts practical significance to the fact that a Locarno formula, if adopted in conditions short of formal agreement on Israeli frontiers in both the east and the west, immediately places Israel in the erstwhile position of France (undertaking to exchange the territorial hold on the Rhineland for the contractual assurance), and the eastern Arabs in that of France's eastern allies (separated and differentiated from their principal ally in the west). Moreover, Locarno will point in the direction of Munich for either the Palestinians or the Israelis objectively and for both subjectively. In such a perspective, the basic principle of a guarantee and its political context and timing are more important than against whom and to what specific performance it commits the United States. Likewise, implications for American and superpower diplomacy, Israeli morale, and American politics are more immediately important than is the proximate military utility of a guarantee.

In order to offset a best-case plaidoyer such as Ullman's, it is legitimate to resort to worst-case arguments. Such arguments leave open the possibility that Kissinger's bag contains a middling nostrum of sorts combining the best—or worst—of both worlds. While we wait for sleights of hand, my basic contention is that a premature guarantee would make the United States into Israel's moral captive while crippling American diplomatic capacity to promote a settlement; it would position Israel for satellite dependence immediately and for graduated compellence and gradual decadence in due course; and it would repolarize the Middle East along lines even less tractable than the current ones.

Clearly, American moral responsibility for Israel grows materially if a guarantee is offered to offset a simultaneous diminution in local capacity for self-defense in still unsettled conditions. Withdrawal from the Sinai passes and, subsequently, in the Golan Heights will so weaken Israel, if to a debatable degree. The consequently enhanced Israeli moral claim can be readily turned into a trigger to set off American performance. A guarantee in any circumstances places Israel in a status loosely comparable with Czechoslovakia's position relative to the French alliance guarantee in the period between Locarno and Munich. Once Israel is deprived or weakened in the "natural" defense frontiers, it begins to combine the attributes of a post-Munich Czechoslovakia that would have received the pledged guarantee to make up for the lost mountainous borders, and of effectively guaranteed Poland taking over from the British the determination as to when their guarantee is to go into effect. The first position is nationally humiliating for the smaller country while the second is internationally explosive. And the parallel is instructive, even when granting the real difference in both guarantor and guaranteed powers.

While in part captive, the United States would be also crippled in both its mediatory diplomacy and its coercive diplomacy. A premature guarantee is apt to "enrage" (Reston's word) the Arabs (including Faisal over Jerusalem, *pace* Ullman) with more radical views and more intractable problems than are Egypt's. Moreover, American capacity for effective pressure on events would be disabled along with evenhandedness. A widely resented interim guarantee would only confirm the Europeans in denying facilities for U.S. military movements to the Middle East. And it would freeze U.S.-Soviet confrontation into a pattern of reflex responses, largely independent of military developments among the local parties to reactivated conflict. An interim U.S. guarantee would not necessarily precipitate an explicit Soviet counter-guarantee. But, insofar as a formalized U.S. commitment created even the presumption of an automatic U.S. performance on Israel's side, it would "guarantee" a reflex Soviet counteraction regardless of prior commitments. Since a *de facto* American guarantee of Israel exists in any event, giving it a juridical form would engender the presumption of automaticity regardless of its actual terms. This is the critical factor. It would tend to eliminate the leverage implicit in an American capacity to merely threaten intervention and in the two superpowers jointly facing the prospect of escalating confrontation, in conditions in which absence of formal commitments matches the absence of a formal settlement.

Far from being built-in, both threat and prospect can be manipulated only in conditions of theoretical choice as the superpowers try to reach a basis for shared restraint or shared responsibility for settlement. It would be unwise, therefore, to exchange a pretended "ambiguity" in the American commitment to Israel (as Ullman would have it) for a spurious certainty injurious to diplomatic flexibility in influencing local parties and bargaining with the Soviet Union. There is no ambiguity to the American commitment in the last resort, and flexibility is essential for all situations short of the sudden imminence of total Israeli defeat. To enclose American statecraft in automatic reflexes would be to write an ironic *finis* to Kissinger's diplomacy of the free hand. Moreover, even supposing that the "certainty" deriving from a U.S. guarantee would deter conventional war without intensifying terroristic violence to fill the consequent vacuum of force, this is unconditionally desirable only if peace-through-peace is viewed as the necessary supplement to peace-by-pieces. Yet to eliminate the war possibility is also to eliminate the still indispensable medium-term leverage for settlement. As leverage, war might still have to intervene somewhere between the failure of both unilateral and multilateral diplomacy and a longer-term (if not necessarily final) politico-military stability under either American-Israeli military or American-Soviet political auspices.

For Israel, a provisional U.S. guarantee for the interim would add little to the defensive security it already derives from the mix of territorial and *de facto* American guarantees. The incremental increase in security would not, therefore, compensate Israel for forfeiting its last-resort preemptive or offensive military option to de-freeze once more the *status quo* for one more try at recasting it for lasting peace. Israel's acceptance of a premature guarantee-cum-withdrawal now would only encourage intransigent Arab parties with a token of Israel's mellowing, to say the least; and it might effectively advance the process of moral decadence. A formally dependent status will psychologically affect any society. In Israel's case, the intangibles might disastrously supplement any long-term relative deterioration in material potential and economic leverage. More immediately significant would be the less hypothetical politico-diplomatic consequence of a premature guarantee tied to a fixed period of time or to visible progress toward political settlement. As time passed without signs of progress on the difficult non-Egyptian issues, the potential of the guarantee for military deterrence would tend to be overshadowed by its potential for graduated political compellence. Pressures on Israel to make concessions would mount even while its capacity to resist them faded at the same increasing rate.

Under the stated circumstances, the only immediate beneficiary of Israeli withdrawal behind the Sinai passes (and from the oil fields) in exchange for a U.S. guarantee that would either replace or supplement Egyptian assurances (to the United States rather than Israel directly) would be Sadat's Egypt or Egypt's Sadat. But even for Sadat, as for Kissinger, the advantage is lastingly worthwhile only if it gives a fresh and decisive impetus to the lagging separate-peace approach toward a general settlement. From the vantage point of the eastern Arabs, a Locarno-type U.S. guarantee prior to a general settlement would be a *de facto* separate, even if only temporary, peace in (the new) place. The key eastern Arab-Israeli frontiers in Syria and cis-Jordan are not only actually controlled by Israel and further vulnerable to it militarily; they are also more controversial than the western ones vis-à-vis Egypt. A Locarno formula applied in the west while controversy continues in the east assimilates the Middle Eastern eastern frontiers to the inter-war Czechoslovak and Polish frontiers with Germany and impliedly certifies them as being second-class relative to the western; and it shields them from forcible change only by paper commitments once the major western military power (France or Egypt, respectively) is precluded from offensive pressure on the strongest central military power (Germany, Israel) in the event of a conflict in the east. The resulting situation would be politically tolerable for Egypt in the Arab world only if Syria and the Palestinians quickly and visibly shared in the benefits; and it would be economically tolerable if the Saudis could register some movement on Jerusalem. Since Egyptian capacity to continue restraint in the west would increasingly depend on Israeli concessions in the east, the pressure on Israel to make such concessions in the interest of the fragile new security system would mount with every Egyptian difficulty. This would more than offset any advantage that Israel might appear to gain from "neutralizing" the principal armed force of the Arab camp.

A separate-peace formula is a time-honored strategy for ending a war which is not total, if the party separated from its allies not only controls the principal assets but is consequently able to carry others into a general settlement willy-nilly. No condition other than conventional military manpower favors a strategy of this kind centered on Egypt. Consequently, a premature Locarno would not unleash a competitive stampede by individual Arab parties for preferential inclusion in the general peace. It would instead tend to repolarize the Middle East along new lines, while intensified sub-conventional warfare would parallel intensified strategic Soviet presence in Syria, Iraq, and possibly elsewhere. Any concurrent diminution of Arab oil money to Egypt could not be compensated by equivalent American donations. Reinforced or rationalized by pan-Arab principles, the resulting economic hardship would stimulate domestic upheaval in Egypt against the new policy. It must be Sadat's current hope, therefore, that his American friend can devise a guarantee formula that, while deterrent to his Israeli adversaries militarily and seductive to them politically, would not be provocative to his Arab allies: a formula that would be stabilizing for him at home and locally while being potentially pacifying all around.

The devising of such formula, if it is indeed being sought for, ought to test the last ingenuity of Kissinger's brilliant lieutenants. Their additional task is to insure that a guarantee formula be also meaningfully additive, or supplemental, to whatever assurances Egypt might privately give to the United States in conditions in which to proffer an American guarantee is to automatically discount the independent value of such private assurances. Only a formula highly executive in kind, elusive in substance, limited in time, and contingent or conditional in its terms can even begin to meet such exacting requirements. Inventing and advancing such a formula might ease Kissinger's immediate problem with the Congress and even impart formal correctitude to the official claim that the guarantee is not a guarantee after all. Yet the more contingent and limited is the guarantee formula, the less is its protective value for Israel and its deterrent value all around, and the less acceptable are, consequently, its diplomatic costs in direct U.S.-Soviet and U.S.-Arab relations.

II

A U.S. security guarantee to Israel, or to Israel and Egypt jointly, in separation from a political settlement would be injurious to both American and Israeli interests and to the cause of permanent peace in the Middle East as well. It is no more in the interest of the United States to slide incrementally into a Middle Eastern guarantee (as the new variant on the step-by-step approach) than it was to slide into the Indochina war. Internally and internationally critical decisions ought to be taken in full cognizance of motives, risks, and as far as possible, circumstances of commitment to military intervention abroad. This is not the time, therefore, to escalate whatever private prior assurances may have been scattered around to facilitate the first disengagement step in Sinai and the Golan Heights. Nor is it in Israel's interest to involve itself in a contractual, Locarno-like net and match America's predicament arising out of nefarious incrementalism with a national disaster due to gradual (moral) decadence and graduated (political) compellence to uncompensated concessions—or to both in different points in time.

If an immediate U.S. guarantee for the interim between the second disengagement step and the final settlement is premature in timing and likely to be prejudicial in its practical bearing, and if the agitation of the guarantee to be part of the final settlement package is likewise premature and may be prejudicial in terms of diplomatic procedure, why the sudden furor? The impression is unavoidable that, in some form, the guarantee phenomenon is a way to keep Kissinger's last step before Geneva from conspicuously failing over the impossibility of Egypt's meeting Syrian and Soviet opposition head on. One can only speculate why it apparently proved impossible to reconcile, in a formula viable for both parties, Kissinger's need for some last face-saving success with the Soviet need to be seen as prevailing over Kissinger's unilateralism at its base while keeping him and his commitment to general détente politically alive by a last superficial concession on the Middle Eastern issue. There can be little doubt that Kissinger's diplomacy required the last success of unilateralism for its prestige more, and more immediately, than either Israel or Egypt needed such success on the grounds of intrinsic merit or as a favorable omen for ultimate achievement in Geneva. If atmospherics was involved, its publicized character along the last-mentioned lines is questionably the main one.

There is little mystery to unravel as regards Kissinger's personal stake as the master diplomatist. Once he effected the delicate transition from airborne shuttle diplomacy to the shores of Lake Geneva, he reached safe haven. If Geneva were to succeed, it would not be possible to convincingly disprove the contention that the prior uni- or bi-lateral preparation was the decisive element; if it were to fail to either edge toward settlement multilaterally or soar toward it on two-power wings, the prior pessimistic Kissinger predictions would stand justified, and the ensuing conflict would reopen the possibility for application of lessons learned from diplomatic mistakes in and after October 1973. The situation is radically different if the last unilateral step to Geneva were to falter. Kissinger needs thus once again overt Israeli and collusive Egyptian help if he is to move forward in appearance at least, and at all costs.

In securing Israeli help, the only direct and immediate coercion available to the Kissinger-Ford team in breaking down Israeli reluctance would be denial of arms. Yet to do so without simultaneously squaring or controlling the Arabs meant always placing the time bomb of consequent Israeli military defeat under U.S. policy externally and U.S. politics internally. This would be all the more true if denial of arms occurred in connection with a package deal (guarantee against withdrawal) that had been recognized as being inimical to the best interests of both Israel and the United States while being deficient in decisive saving features relative to the Arab or Soviet sides. The threat of arms denial is empty when it is not counterproductive in that peculiar context: the fewer arms Israel receives, the sooner will this activate the clock on the time bomb and concurrently bring into play the *de facto* U.S. guarantee of ultimate Israeli territorial integrity and political independence. To revive for the last time the inter-war analogy, no U.S. government could credibly follow vis-à-vis Israel in the steps of the French and British governments when they threatened to abandon Czechoslovakia to its fate if it refused to comply with their advice to surrender defensible strategic frontiers in all circumstances or in the absence of equivalent security. This limitation on American statecraft in the Middle East may have been regrettable in the past and may again become so; it is currently a desirable check on the vagaries of a too-personal diplomacy.

The reason is that Kissinger's Middle Eastern diplomacy is not wholly identifiable with American foreign policy for the area. What is or might be a catastrophe for Kissinger's diplomacy personally might be only a setback or even a platform for American policy if it were to pass into other hands. While the United States would still go to Geneva under the cloud of the failure to extrude

the Soviet Union and bring lasting peace in the Middle East single-
handedly, the clouds would lift rapidly as the Soviets sought to
reestablish a détente threatened by the departure of its American
embodiment and to do so on new and possibly more reliable foundations that would profitably include movement toward superpower accord for the Middle East. Alternatively, the Arab parties
themselves would seek to offset too great an initial Soviet advantage and U.S. disadvantage by moving to the American side as part
of their inveterate balancing approach to politics. At the very least,
an American diplomacy freed from personal commitment to the
unilateral approach and unburdened by predictions of failure at
Geneva would be better able to project the image of basic American good faith in giving Geneva a fair try. This might be important
domestically as well if the failure in Geneva were to be a prelude
to one more war in the Middle East. As part of such a war, a new
secretary of state might still be able to learn from Kissinger's
misjudgments during and following the October war without inject-
ing a frustrated ego into the delicate and possibly explosive exercise in superpower confrontational diplomacy that such correction
might well entail.

On the theory of negotiating while fighting, which is a theory
shared by classic and communist statecraft, it is possible to argue
that even the first disengagement undermined the progress toward
political settlement by removing the pressure of an "untenable"
military situation from the "intractable" character of the politico-
territorial issues left to themselves. From a more prudent viewpoint, the first-step disengagement in Egypt and Syria made sense
in determining whether the politico-territorial issues could be re-
solved (with American assistance) outside the framework of a
U.S.-Soviet confrontation or "condominium" (or, in succession,
both) within a time frame that would not materially change the
existing local balances of power. When the predictably negative
answer began to emerge, the continued pursuit of the mirage of a
self-amplifying separate-peace arrangement with Egypt decayed
quickly into a search for ever new gestures of good will while
reducing real incentives for the local parties to show effective will
for good (i.e., permanent peace). This was most particularly true
for the parties that were getting a little more each time in the short
run and had everything to hope for in an open-ended long run. The

critical issue was then whether it would be the non-Egyptian Arabs or Israel that would be drawn into a final-peace situation, even if not a formal settlement, while under a sufficiently prolonged spell of the absence of mind: the last best hope of any gradualist approach to major structural political problems. To say so much is to argue that if the first step in the Middle East was potentially useful —even if only for exploratory purposes—the second step currently at issue has been in no convincing way necessary for the final settling of the truly difficult questions when one discounts the psychological good-will factor in relation to the eastern Arabs and questions the possible momentum of the separate-peace strategy centered on Egypt.

The frail present hope must be for a Geneva miracle to take over from the Kissinger magic in resolving the difficult questions while Israel can still wait for reasons of regional and overall international balance of material power and the Arab governments can still wait for domestic political reasons. If there is no evidence of a meaningful progress, the role of Geneva will rapidly become for diplomatic strategy what the role of the initial disengagements was for military tactics: to set or define the starting positions for a next round of fighting. Through the conference the small-state parties will start seeking alibis as powers that had war "imposed" upon them by the other side's intransigence. In the best of cases, the superpowers will seek alibis with the small powers for "imposing" a political settlement on the prospective belligerents. They will do so if they (or only the more reluctant Soviet Union?) decide to have the concert-condominium formula in effect imposed upon themselves by the prospect of intolerable confrontation, and possibly direct involvement, in a truly serious next (and "last"?) round of fighting as the alternative.

Such a round would respond to qualitatively different imperatives from the earlier ones. The oil issue, as part of these, may strengthen Israel's position militarily to compensate for having weakened it previously in the politico-economic realm. Moreover, the oil issue will also predictably affect the superpower politics of confrontation. It will strengthen the Soviet reluctance to see the United States have its way with the Arabs for economic reasons as a matter of overt superpower competition even while reinforcing the American entitlement to resist "strangulation" as part of the tacit superpower accord—or rules of the game—barring major one-shot setback or deprivation from preexisting conditions for either of the two major players.

III

A next round of fighting in the Middle East consequent on a failure at Geneva would differ from past ones also (if not only) by combining the Arab-Israeli issue with the oil issue. As the two aspects merge, different scenarios—entailing different choices for the United States—can be envisioned.

Reasonable Arab governments, if they can withstand popular pressure for an oil embargo while Arab armies hold their own with Israel, or are winning over Israel, will in principle prefer not to give the United States gratuitously the strangulation pretext for a military intervention reinforcing the Israeli side. But in the postulated case of a stalemate or Israeli setbacks, the United States will have an incentive to intensify military aid to Israel and an excuse for involvement that *could* be extended to deal with the oil issue's long-term impact on Western economies. The mere possibility or anticipation of such American reactions might induce even reluctant Arab governments to use their ultimate oil weapon preemptively, in the hope perhaps of bringing pressure to bear on the United States via the more sensitive European and Japanese economies. Alternatively, on the analogy of the suicidal nuclear spasm, the Arabs could impose the embargo as the last-resort reflex response to a crushing military defeat. A simultaneously unfolding major Israeli victory would provide a basis for a U.S. response that could be only indirect: i.e., holding the ring so as to impede or prevent a correcting Soviet intervention on the Arab side. The premise behind that merely indirect approach would be that a decisive Israeli victory would weaken or eliminate the oil pressure by the strain a major or "decisive" defeat would place on the internal cohesion of the Arab component of OPEC—and thus bring the latter to disintegration.

Concurrently, an unchecked Israeli victory would set the stage for a political settlement for at least a medium term on the basis of either a reinstated Israeli military hegemony regionally, at once underwritten and contained by the United States, or, as the only available alternative to it from the Soviet and Arab viewpoints, a U.S.-Soviet solution on an equilibrium basis that would be differently favorable to Israel and might be longer-lasting. An equilibrium "solution" on less-favorable terms to Israel could also follow upon one more Israeli-Arab military stalemate, or even a moderate Israeli military setback, that the superpowers would manage differently from last time. In such a situation, a simultaneous American military implantation in the Persian Gulf oil fields or in the Mediterranean littoral would be an additional bargaining counter on the U.S.-Israeli side. The actually transpired scenario could thus be a modified Suez of 1956: direct introduction of U.S. (or Western) forces in the Middle East, but now in the context of Arab-Israeli stalemate or Israeli setback. Or it could be a new Cuba: U.S. "victory" in a nuclear confrontation with the Soviet Union on the basis of both local conventional and general "procedural" advantages (Israel's success in the field and a superior American capacity for invading the oil fields, and—on the procedural side—a better American "title" arising from the reciprocally acknowledged right to superpower self-defense extended henceforth to matters economic).

In the first scenario, a direct U.S. intervention against the embargo in the Persian Gulf or in Libya would be tactically disjoined from the Arab-Israeli conflict and only strategically complementary with it. In the second, an indirect U.S. military involvement via deterrent confrontation with the Soviet Union would have only a coincidental strategic impact on the oil issue alongside a crushing Israeli military success and only supportive tactical consequences on the ground (by impeding the Soviet Union from strengthening the Arabs). But, under either of the scenarios, the United States would be acting indistinguishalby as both a NATO power (in defense of Western Europe and Japan with their consent and support, or in spite of them) and as an *ad hoc* Middle Eastern power. American capacity to act militarily—i.e., using European NATO bases, etc.—would be materially increased if a prior oil embargo gave direct justification; European consent in any circumstances would be facilitated if American will and ability to act effectively were beyond reasonable doubt. In the best of all possible alliance worlds, or in the worst of possible economic emergencies, it might even prove possible to improvise some kind of joint U.S.-European operation, if only to remove the European fears of the hegemonial implications of Europe being "saved" once again by the United States unaided. In the absence of direct Arab economic threat, European cooperation or tolerance would be less certain. But cooperation would be at least marginally improved if the Arab side had not been previously politically provoked by a premature or prior guarantee to Israel and if the Geneva conference had failed without any traceable U.S. responsibility for that failure.

In due course, the possibility of a joint or parallel U.S. and Soviet guarantee in the Middle East will have to be placed seriously on the agenda, as either an alternative to continuing underhanded competition or a remedy to recurrent dramatic confrontations. Any such effort will probably signal the failure of routine unilateral or multilateral diplomatic procedures seeking to remove the Arab-Israeli settlement from the context of both local force and U.S.-Soviet power, or it might be the real basis of a Geneva settlement underneath a multilateral façade. Following the stage when "imposition" of settlement by the superpowers was pronounced morally unthinkable, it is now merely discounted as politically unfeasible. Such an impossibility is, however, only an unexamined premise as long as it is not seriously tested at all, is fallaciously tested to provide an alibi for forcing a Soviet strategic retreat from the area (as was in part at least the case in October 1973), or is only half-heartedly tested in most unfavorable circumstances (e.g., reportedly, by Ford and Kissinger while unilateralism faltered in the Middle East, while the situation there was relatively relaxed militarily, and while détente was under stress from invalid alternative testing by senatorial diplomacy in its economic dimension). The attraction of an American-Soviet accord in the Middle Est will, however, persist as long as there is interest in a stable Middle East and, concurrently, in a security setting within which Israel can safely accept contractual guarantees in exchange for territorial insurance and within which the United States can underwrite Israeli security without automatically favoring the Soviets with some at least of the oil-producing Arabs.

The methods for implementing the accord by way of an American-Soviet guarantee of a permanent settlement can be explored hypothetically even while the realization is not imminent practically. Only one thing seems certain: to either introduce an interim guarantee now, or to finalize by congressional or any other official U.S. action the terms of a one-sided American guarantee as the prospective part of a permanent settlement, and only subsequently to invite the Soviets to join in such a guarantee, would be one more exercise in unilateralism almost certain to fulfill the underlying expectation of a Soviet refusal. The exercise would only replay, under quite different circumstances and for less legitimate reasons, the American "invitation" to the Soviet Union to join in the Marshall Plan for stabilization in the then-troubled Europe—an invitation which, at the time, actually intensified the contest over spheres of influence that has only now, largely on Soviet terms, resulted in a superstructure of European "security and cooperation" engaging both superpowers along with the local parties.

In a "final" settlement which does not coincide with expelling the Soviet Union from the Middle East (and, consequently, with a U.S.-sponsored Israeli military predominance or regional politico-economic equilibrium), an American guarantee could be matched by a parallel but non-competitive Soviet guarantee of its Arab protégés or be comprised in a joint U.S.-Soviet guarantee of the Locarno type for the entire Middle East. A joint U.S.-Soviet guarantee would mean in practice that the special entrenchment of each superpower in its sphere of influence has also a condominial superstructure. Either format is consistent with a settlement in some way "imposed" by the superpowers. When Kissinger says, as his senior journalistic confidant and *porte-parole*[3] reports, "if we go to Geneva without an agreement beforehand, you will know that no agreement is possible," the statement, to be exact, would have to continue: "[impossible] by virtue of unilateral American efforts and on the basis of a spontaneous choice of local parties." There *is* an agreement about *what* should be settled at Geneva or elsewhere, Reston's belief to the contrary. What is not agreed is *how* it ought to be settled and, especially, *by whom*.

From the U.S. viewpoint, more important than the specific form of Soviet participation in guarantee is the area and extent of Soviet post-settlement entrenchment. The basic question is: Will legitimizing the Soviet presence solidify it and thus moderate its reach,

---

[3] James Reston, "Guarantee for Israel?" *New York Times*, February 21, 1975, p. 31.

while the lessened Arab needs for Soviet arms and military instruction against Israel reduce Soviet capacity for complete takeover in
any one country? For the Soviets themselves, two basic quandaries
arise. First, ought they to collaborate in settling the too-explosive
Arab-Israeli conflict on the assumption that the consequently intensified conflicts among Arab or Islamic powers (e.g., Iraq versus
Kuwait, Iran, or Saudi Arabia) will continue local needs for Soviet
support in a restructured neither-war-nor-peace situation, initially
safer in terms of superpower relations and susceptible of extending
via Pakistan and India into the Indian Ocean area with a potentially positive anti-Chinese potential? Secondly, if the answer is
affirmative, ought the Soviets prefer to diffuse their influence as co-
guarantors more widely (to encompass Israel among others) or
hope to concentrate the influence more deeply as but parallel
guarantors?

As for Israel, it may come to prefer a joint U.S.-Soviet guarantee for the Middle East on the assumption that it would reduce
political dependence on the U.S.; would dilute the American safeguard only negligibly if at all, even if performance under the joint
guarantee were to be contingent on Soviet co-determination or
actual participation in enforcement; and would not materially expand the risks of Soviet intrusion in internal Israeli affairs. A basic
consideration tipping the balance of such particular cost-benefit
calculations might well bear on the question of whether Israel
ought to compensate for the reduction in status from a regionally
hegemonial to a globally protected small state in the typical equilibrium fashion of the small state, i.e., by finding all sorts of advantages (and risks) in counterpoising one great power against another.

It is not in the long-term Israeli interest, now or after settlement,
to be identified with the United States as either the virtual fifty-first
state of the union or the cat's-paw of American imperialism. Nor is
such identification to the advantage of American domestic or global politics, unless it becomes the only viable formula for regional
stability in the medium term. It would become so only after the
United States had failed to secure an "evenhanded" solution for
the region's small states by means of a vigorous—but not high-
handed—diplomatic procedure with respect to the Soviet Union.
Such a failure would place U.S. policy under the strain of having to

provide against long-term deterioration of Israel's material position regionally and its diplomatic position globally. The strain would be considerable, since that very failure would reflect, and might accentuate, a progressive decline in the global position of the U.S. itself. Inefficacy in the Middle East would tend to characterize the United States conclusively as a nation too-easily disposed to seek refuge from immediate risks of militarily encompassed tragedy in a pathetic alliance with regionally declining states: as a country unwilling and unable to revive its impaired credibility as a world power capable of decisive intervention even in an area where, under proper circumstances, it can count on sufficient domestic support and solid economic rationale.

One precondition of this support would be that the Arabs had conclusively rejected—while the Israelis had gone far toward conceding—a settlement on the basis of the military stalemate of 1973 which restored the Arabs' military honor; and that the Soviet Union had turned its back upon a settlement that would place it near both political parity in the Middle East and coequal status as a world power. The other condition would be that the United States was reentering the military arena by deliberate choice, with congressional sanction, on the basis of at least initially known circumstances, and for reasons and from motives which would neither extend personal commitments nor react to personal frustrations. If this country is not to find Kissinger's peace by straightforward progression along his chosen path, let it by all means not have Kissinger's war in the Middle East in circumstances reminiscent of McNamara's and Johnson's war in Southeast Asia.

LIBRARY OF CONGRESS CATALOGING IN PUBLICATION DATA

Liska, George.
  Beyond Kissinger.

  Bibliography: p.
    1. Diplomacy. 2. Kissinger, Henry Alfred. 3. United States—For-
eign relations—1945–   I. Title. II. Series: Washington Center of
Foreign Policy Research. Studies in international affairs; no. 26)
JX1662.L56   327'.2'0973   75–10838

ISBN 0–8018–1763–3
ISBN 0–8018–1764–1 pbk.